Medical Ethics and the Elderly

THIRD EDITION

Edited by
GURCHARAN S RAI
Consultant Physician, Whittington Hospital, London
Honorary Senior Lecturer, Royal Free and
University College Medical School, London

Forewords by
JEREMY PLAYFER AND MARSHALL B KAPP

Law sections edited by
GURDEEP S RAI

Cartoons by
IVA BLACKMAN

Radcliffe Publishing
Oxford • New York

Radcliffe Publishing Ltd
18 Marcham Road
Abingdon
Oxon OX14 1AA
United Kingdom

www.radcliffe-oxford.com

Electronic catalogue and worldwide online ordering facility.

First Edition 1999 (published by Taylor & Francis)
Second Edition 2004

British Library Cataloguing in Publication Data

A catalogue record for this book is available from the British Library.

ISBN-13: 978 184619 307 1

The paper used for the text pages of this book
is FSC certified. FSC (The Forest Stewardship
Council) is an international network to promote
responsible management of the world's forests.

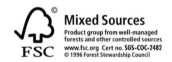

Mixed Sources
Product group from well-managed
forests and other controlled sources
www.fsc.org Cert no. SGS-COC-2482
© 1996 Forest Stewardship Council

FSC

Typeset by Pindar NZ, Auckland, New Zealand
Printed and bound by TJI Digital, Padstow, Cornwall, UK

Medical Ethics and the Elderly

Contents

Preface to the third edition

Since the publication of the second edition, the Mental Capacity Act 2005 received Royal Assent in 2005 and was implemented in two stages in 2007. This Act provides a comprehensive framework for decision making on behalf of adults who lack capacity to make decisions on their own behalf. In addition, there have been several other significant publications including:

- an update on consent from the General Medical Council in 2008
- a guide from the National Council for Palliative Care on advance decisions to refuse treatment
- a British Medical Association publication on end-of-life decisions in 2007
- guidance from the National Institute for Health and Clinical Excellence and the Social Care Institute for Excellence on supporting people with dementia and their carers in health and social care in 2006
- an update on decisions relating to cardiopulmonary resuscitation from the British Medical Association in 2007
- new guidance on confidentiality from the General Medical Council in 2004
- National Health Service Code of Practice on Confidentiality in 2005.

The updated chapters have included the provisions of the Mental Capacity Act and the above publications. In addition, we have included a new chapter on communication with older people. However, the main aim of the book remains the same – it is intended to be a practical guide for junior medical staff, including specialist registrars. Other professionals who are involved with doctors in making difficult decisions will also find this text useful, as will medical students who now have to learn about medical ethics and their application in day-to-day management of patients, as part of the undergraduate curriculum.

Gurcharan S Rai
May 2009

Preface to the second edition

Since the publication of the first edition of this book in 1999 we have seen the introduction of the Human Rights Act 1998, which incorporates the European Convention of Human Rights into UK law, the production of new guidelines on cardiopulmonary resuscitation by the British Medical Association in 2002, the new draft bill on mental incapacity, the new guidelines on consent for treatment and the publication of the National Service Framework for Older People, with a commitment to abolish ageism in clinical practice. The updated chapters have included these changes in law, the new guidelines and the new standards set out in the National Service Framework for Older People. In addition, two important new chapters on confidentiality and on ethical issues and driving have been added.

However, the main aim of the book remains the same – it is intended to be a practical guide for junior medical staff, including specialist registrars. Other professionals who are involved with doctors in making difficult decisions will also find this text useful, as will medical students who now have to learn about medical ethics and their application in day-to-day management of patients, as part of the undergraduate curriculum.

Gurcharan S Rai
March 2004

Foreword

Ten years in print and a new third edition of *Medical Ethics and the Elderly* is a cause for celebration. The book takes its place in the canon of Geriatric Medicine, earned because of its relevance and clear presentation of the complex moral issues. The third edition is reinvigorated by the addition of new younger authors who have upheld the tradition of concise incisive contributions informed by active engagement with clinical problems. The book retains its shape, style and length, resisting the temptation to expand the content beyond recognition. There is only one additional chapter 'Communication, barriers to it and information sharing' which is well written and thought provoking. Dr Gurcharan Rai has shown great skill in editing, incorporating the many changes in legislation that have occurred since the second edition while retaining the practicality and instructiveness of the text.

Medical ethics continues to grow in importance as a core subject in medical education. Those of us dealing with the old and vulnerable need to have skills in ethical reasoning and an up-to-date knowledge of the relevant legislation. This book more than achieves its aims of providing not only a practical guide but also a readable account of the principles and practice of ethics as they apply to the specialty of medicine for the elderly. It can be used both for reference and as a textbook from which the basic skills of ethical reasoning can be acquired. A must read book for anyone training in the specialty and an essential core text for every geriatrician's office.

The ethical challenges the medical profession face are becoming more demanding. The developments of high-tech interventions pose both benefits and risks to patients. The public are thankfully better informed and able to exert more influence on issues which were previously reserved to professionals. For example, there is a growing clamour for physician-assisted suicide in terminally ill patients which divides professional opinion. Doctors need to be able to react to the challenges in an informed professional manner that can only be achieved by them having the ethical literacy which is exemplified by the contents of this excellent book.

Doctors like certainty and medicine is easy when one can make decisions by simply following guidelines or protocols. Geriatrics is however probably the most complex branch of medicine. Most of our decisions fall in the grey area between black and white. In trying to make the best choices for patients, ethical considerations always play a part. Dr Gurchuran Rai exemplifies a careful and thoughtful approach to medicine and his achievement in editing three editions of this influential book, including his own original contributions, is to be greatly admired.

I unreservedly recommend this book. The new edition meets the requirements of today's practice and this and future editions will provide a core text for doctors and students for many years to come.

Jeremy Playfer MD FRCP
Emeritus Consultant, Royal Liverpool
and Broadgreen University Hospital
Honorary Clinical Lecturer, University of Liverpool
and Past President, British Geriatrics Society
May 2009

Foreword

Since publication of the second edition of this book in 2004, the international phenomenon of rapid population aging has continued unabated. Similarly, the medical, ethical, legal, social and economic challenges accompanying this demographic development have grown, and continue to grow, increasingly numerous and complex. For example, in the United Kingdom over the past half decade, a panoply of legislative developments (including receipt of Royal Assent to The Mental Capacity Act in 2005) and organisational guidelines and codes pertaining to the ethical delivery of medical care to older individuals have emerged and are reflected in many parts of this new third edition.

Similarly, there has been a great amount of relevant legal and economic activity in recent years in the United States in response to the graying of its citizenry. Of course, important differences persist between the UK and the United States in terms of legal, social and economic climate, and those differences certainly may affect the ethics of providing – and paying for – healthcare for older persons in each country.

Nonetheless, there remain important commonalities in the basic values and tensions confronting medical caregivers for the aged in both nations. Generic ethical concerns that UK and American healthcare providers regularly confront (such as the need to delicately balance moral reverence for individual self-determination, on one hand, and society's simultaneous responsibility to maximise the older person's good and minimise harm, on the other) may be characterised by unique nuances in the geriatric arena. The special challenges involved in caring for the aged may result from particular factors inherent in this patient population (for example, a higher incidence and prevalence of cognitive and emotional impairment), the types of institutional and community settings within which geriatric services are provided, and the focus of geriatric care on the objectives of maximising the patient's ability to function well in daily life and achieve an optimal quality of life, rather than on simply extending the length of life.

In both the UK and the US, ethical decisions must be made and actions taken (or purposefully not taken) within distinct legal boundaries. Despite the legal superstructure in each jurisdiction, however, the ethical aspects of medical care remain for the most part self-enforcing. Thus, the various chapters in this book acknowledge that geriatric practice 'on the ground' (that is, in real life situations) is determined by healthcare provider virtues and patient wishes as much, if not more, than by academic ethics or legal edicts emanating from the legislature, government agency, or the judiciary.

This comprehensive and timely third edition should assist geriatric professionals to manage, in an ethically tolerable and perhaps even laudatory manner, circumstances entailing inconsistent and sometimes seemingly incompatible individual and institutional values. The chapter contributors do not pretend that there are objectively 'correct' answers to the dilemmas posed by an aging patient population, but they do make available to the reader – through the skillful employment of numerous hypothetical problems, among other effective methods of presentation – a very useful grounding upon which to build more-than-adequate applied ethical analyses of key concerns.

Differences in legal, social and economic climates notwithstanding, there is much that the UK and US aging services communities can teach to, and learn from, each other. Even more than its previous version, this thoroughly updated edition of *Medical Ethics and the Elderly* will not only assist physicians, medical students, and other healthcare providers in the UK regarding the ethical questions with which they regularly must deal, but will also facilitate cross-national pollination of ethical ideas and skills among healthcare practitioners on both sides of the Atlantic.

Marshall B Kapp JD, MPH, FCLM
Garwin Distinguished Professor of Law and Medicine
Southern Illinois University School of Law, USA
May 2009

About the editor

Gurcharan S Rai is consultant physician at the Whittington Hospital, London, and is a member of the British Geriatrics Society and of its Special Group on Medical Ethics, and a Fellow of the American Geriatrics Society. He has extensive experience in the teaching and training of undergraduates and postgraduates and at the present time is Chair of the Training Committee and Regional Adviser for Geriatric Medicine in North Thames (East).

List of contributors

Jonathan Birns
Consultant in Stroke Medicine, Geriatrics and General Medicine
Guy's & St Thomas' NHS Foundation Trust

Iva Blackman
Consultant Physician and Geriatrician

Ann Bowling
Professor of Health Services Research
University College London

Sally Briggs
Specialist Registrar in Geriatric and General Internal Medicine
North Western Deanery

Jim Eccles
Consultant Physician in Geriatric Medicine
St James' University Hospital, Leeds

Philippa Gee
Highly Specialist Speech and Language Therapist
Royal Berkshire NHS Foundation Trust, Reading

Catherine Harvey
Consultant in Care of Elderly and Acute Medicine
University College London Hospital

Steven Luttrell
Consultant Physician in Older People's Services
St Pancras Hospital
Medical Director
Camden Primary Care Trust

David Oliver
Professor of Medicine for Older People
City University, London

Desmond O'Neill
Associate Professor
Department of Gerontology, Trinity Centre for Health Sciences
Adelaide and Meath Hospital, Dublin

Kamilla K Porter
Sessional General Practitioner
Southend-on-Sea

Gurdeep S Rai
Solicitor

David Robinson
Associate Professor
Department of Gerontology, Trinity Centre for Health Sciences
Adelaide and Meath Hospital, Dublin

Gwen M Sayers
Consultant Physician London

Kevin Stewart
Consultant Geriatrician
Royal Hampshire County Hospital, Winchester

Martin J Vernon
Consultant Physician in Elderly Medicine
Wythenshawe Hospital, Manchester

Acknowledgement

Most of the chapters in this book contain information on the Mental Capacity Act 2005. It is acknowledged that information on it, particularly in Chapter 5 comes from the Mental Capacity Act of Code of Practice, Issued by the Lord Chancellor on 23 April 2007 in accordance with sections 42 and 43 of the Mental Capacity Act 2005 and published by Department for Constitutional Affairs, London TSO (The Stationery Office).

CHAPTER 1

Principles of medical ethics

Kamilla K Porter and Gurcharan S Rai

Medical knowledge and technology have advanced at a spectacular rate. This voyage of discovery has led to a wealth of ethical issues unimaginable to the original followers of the Hippocratic oath. Steeped in the history of philosophy and religion, the development of medical ethics has been an attempt to unravel and resolve the moral complexities and dilemmas that have faced doctors through the ages. Several tenets of medical ethics have survived to the modern day – for example, *primum non nocere* (first do no harm). Other concepts, such as the notion of communal responsibility and justice, have arisen in the complex modern medical era. What the twenty-first century medical practitioner requires is a comprehensive framework to help identify and critically reflect upon ethical problems.

There are four widely accepted general principles of medical ethics which go towards such a framework, namely autonomy, justice, beneficence and non-maleficence. This 'four-principle' model of moral principles central to biomedical ethics was pioneered by the ethicists Beauchamp and Childress.[1] This approach has met with some criticism as being too simplistic, but of great appeal is that these prima facie principles offer flexibility, represent a neutral frame of reference applicable to patients from different cultures and religions and are independent of political doctrines.[2] There has been a proliferation of ethical guidelines from different medical professional bodies such as the General Medical Council (GMC) and medical defence organisations with regard to clinical practice as well as local and national ethical codes with regard to research. In addition, the 1998 Human Rights Act has had an impact on ethical decisions in the setting of healthcare. For example, Article 2 (right to life), Article 3 (right to freedom from inhuman and degrading treatment) and Article 14 (right to be free from discriminatory practices such as ageism) will affect policies relating to resuscitation orders, aspects of palliative care practice and the level of care in nursing homes.[3]

The profile of patient autonomy has also been raised further as the media and the Internet have provided the public with greater access to information on medicine and health. The 'four-principle' approach discussed in this introductory chapter does not serve as a manual with precise instructions, but rather it provides a framework with which to analyse ethical problems and guidelines. A useful way of thinking about the four-principle model is to consider each principle as one of the four nucleotides that constitute 'moral DNA', capable in combination or on their own of clarifying and justifying the general norms that underlie healthcare ethics.[4]

AUTONOMY

Autonomy is about respecting patients' wishes and facilitating and encouraging their input into the medical decision-making process. The issue of informed consent and refusal lies at the heart of this principle. To respect a patient's autonomy is to give that individual a greater balance of power in the doctor–patient relationship. It entails explaining not only what is wrong with that person, but also the options and implications of any proposed investigation and treatment and the associated risks and benefits. The practitioner needs to provide the patient with as much information as he or she both wishes for and requires in order to make a decision.

Such information needs to be delivered in a clear and concise manner. A balance must be struck between confusing the individual with medical jargon and adopting an overly simplified approach that fails to include important details. The art of pitching the consultation at the right level is by no means straightforward, but where possible by ensuring that the patient understands his or her particular medical problem and management options the doctor should avoid the pitfall of using his or her own personal value system to judge what is best for the patient.

The issue of autonomy is all the more poignant among the elderly population in a society where older people can lose respect and personal choice. With its emphasis on patient-centred care and rooting out age discrimination, the National Service Framework for Older People is promoting greater autonomy among the elderly, highlighting 'the need to view service users as active participants in, rather than subjects of, the care-providing process'.[5]

The application of the principle of autonomy can be seen in the following case of an 80-year-old diabetic woman who was admitted to hospital with cardiac failure following a myocardial infarction. Her mental faculties were fully intact and she was making a steady recovery when her foot became ischaemic. Conservative management was instigated, but the foot could not be salvaged. The vascular surgeons explained on several occasions that in order to curtail the ascending ischaemia and to prevent potentially life-threatening infection, she needed a below-knee amputation. She was informed of her considerable anaesthetic risk, as well as the likelihood of remaining in hospital for several weeks after surgery and then needing a substantial care package. The patient requested time to talk to her family, and after further discussion with both the physicians and surgeons she declined surgery. Over the ensuing days her leg became gangrenous and she died from overwhelming sepsis. The case sparked differing viewpoints among the medical staff, some of whom felt that with the option of local anaesthetic block instead of a general anaesthetic, it was worth risking surgery to prevent this hitherto active and independent individual dying from sepsis. Others felt that with dedicated nursing care and good pain control, the patient's refusal to go ahead with surgery was preferable to a long and complicated recovery period and loss of her independent lifestyle.

This case scenario illustrates how, when management options are no longer clear-cut, the patient can play a pivotal role in guiding the doctor through an ethical maze. The principle of autonomy, although a noble ideal, is not without its limitations. Patients may be unable to contribute fully to discussions about their care for a variety of reasons – for example, in an emergency situation when swift intervention is needed, or when there are communication difficulties which could be due to cultural and language barriers or practical problems such as impairment after a stroke. Furthermore, some patients may reject opportunities to exercise their autonomy and request that the doctor acts on their behalf, as is evident in the statement 'whatever you think best, doctor'. Under such circumstances the doctor may have to decide on the most appropriate course of action, but only after they have given that patient the option of sharing in the decision-making process.

Doctors themselves may feel threatened and challenged by involving patients in making decisions about treatment – for example, due to time constraints in a busy clinic or surgery and a lack of appropriate information to support patients' decisions. Some doctors may feel uncomfortable and lack the skills to negotiate a decision with the patient.[6] This is an area of ongoing research and one which has implications for medical training. It has been argued that failing to accommodate patients' needs and preferences will ultimately diminish doctors' standing.[7]

Respecting autonomy becomes more complicated in cases of mental incompetence. Deciding how to treat the elderly woman with the ischaemic foot would have been more difficult if she had also been suffering from dementia. In such situations the doctor is obliged to look beyond the individual in the sick bed and to consider the patient in the context of her home and family – in other words, taking into account quality-of-life issues. Other health professionals, family members and carers can provide invaluable information. The patient may have made her wishes clear to relatives before her mental deterioration, or appointed an attorney under the lasting power of attorney or in the form of a living will or advance refusal/advance directive. The ethical reverberations of mental incompetence and the issues of living wills, advance decision and quality-of-life measurements are examined in detail in later chapters.

JUSTICE

In the context of healthcare, justice implies an impartial and fair approach to treatment and the distribution of resources. Doctors discriminate unfairly if they allow their prejudices to directly influence their professional work. Established ethical and human rights codes condemn any form of discrimination on the grounds of age, race, sex, religion or sexual orientation. A much-debated topic is whether to continue to provide unrestricted healthcare to individuals whose lifestyle choices and behaviour have contributed to their ill health, for example smoking, intravenous drug use and obesity. If, despite appropriate advice and information about the dangers of high-risk activities such as smoking, a patient continues to take that risk, accepting their decision is effectively taking into account that patient's autonomy. At the same time, encouraging the patient to take responsibility for their medical problems is also to respect their autonomy. Recently published guidance by the GMC on personal beliefs and medical practice stresses that doctors must not allow any personal views about patients to prejudice their assessment of the patient's clinical needs or delay or restrict their access to care.

However, as the cost of healthcare continues to spiral, the issue of social justice and the needs of other health service users cannot be overlooked. Would it be fair to withhold treatment for those who engage in voluntary risk taking at the expense of their health? There are no easy answers to this question, and it is difficult to attribute an individual's ill health solely to their personal actions, as genetic, environmental and social factors can also play a role. Furthermore, some risk taking can result in less rather than more healthcare costs, as such individuals may die earlier and more quickly than those who engage in a less risky lifestyle.[8]

A caring society demands that limited resources are allocated in a just manner. The *Oxford Dictionary of Philosophy* defines distributive justice as 'the link between a distributive system and the maximisation of well-being'. Difficulties arise because of the inevitable scarcity of resources and subsequent conflicts between competing specialty groups. Increasingly, health professionals and governments are confronted with legitimate competing concerns and are having to acknowledge the prioritisation of patient needs. When a potential treatment is wanted for a patient, the final decision may be that due to the overwhelming need of others, the purchasing of this expensive treatment cannot be justified. Numerous national and local clinical guidelines have emerged in recent years. These do not necessarily take the sting out of the tail when an individual's requests are denied – consider the outcry over the National Institute for Health and Clinical Excellence (NICE) guidance for use of acetylcholinesterase inhibiting drugs in the treatment of Alzheimer's disease. A difficult balance has to be struck between personal autonomy and the benefit to society at large.

In an era of increasing healthcare costs, an ageing population and development of more sophisticated treatments and procedures, the issue of healthcare rationing cannot be avoided. Central to this issue are questions of what we mean by human dignity and what level of basic care can still be deemed humane. Setting and defining the limits of an acceptable level of minimum medical care is a dynamic process that requires input from medical professionals, politicians, health managers and the general public. It has been argued that at the very least the aim of basic healthcare is to prevent premature death, to enable an individual to function as a productive member of society and, when that is no longer possible, to alleviate distressing symptoms for the remaining duration of that individual's life and as he or she approaches death.[9]

BENEFICENCE AND NON-MALEFICENCE

The doctor should act to promote the welfare of his or her patient and to do good (beneficence). An action that is taken to benefit the patient may entail risks, so at the same time we have to consider the principle of non-maleficence (avoiding doing harm). In essence we are looking at a cost–benefit ratio, and it is of critical importance that it is patient centred. Acting in the best interests of the patient is a stance that also incorporates respecting autonomy, and conflicts can arise between these principles. Consider the patient who requests an investigation or treatment which the doctor finds to be unwarranted clinically – for example, a lumbar spine X-ray for an episode of mild lower back pain. The doctor's refusal could be seen as paternalistic, and the patient may feel aggrieved, but the doctor has to weigh up the risks and merits of the intervention requested against the patient's wishes and the preservation of a good doctor–patient relationship.

Sometimes the risk of harm to others in the population needs to be taken into account, and the principle of non-maleficence may outweigh the patient's autonomy. An example would be the detention in hospital of a patient who has pulmonary tuberculosis and has repeatedly failed to take their medication regularly in the community. Such drastic action has been deemed ethical on the grounds of the infective risk that the patient poses to the public, and the possibility that he could develop multi-drug resistance and become more unwell through his haphazard use of medication.

Deciding what is beneficial overall to the patient and what constitutes harm can be fraught with difficulty, particularly with regard to end-of-life decisions such as withholding or withdrawing treatment and the much-debated issue of euthanasia and physician-assisted suicide. The notion of saving life underpins medical training. However, nowadays there is also a greater emphasis on examining the quality of life and the concept of dignified death. In the UK, where euthanasia is illegal, doctors follow the doctrine of double effect, under which it is permissible to administer medication to alleviate distressing symptoms of terminal illness even though the patient may die sooner as a result, but the doctor has to prove that the objective is to relieve suffering, not to shorten life. The fear is that if doctors actively assisted patients in ending their lives, the door would be opened to a slippery slope towards involuntary euthanasia where the old or frail might be put under pressure by relatives or be made to feel like an unwanted burden to their families and society. Some argue that there is a very thin line between respecting a terminally ill patient's refusal of life-sustaining treatment and yet turning down their request for assistance in directly ending their life in order to avoid more suffering.[10] These topics will be explored further in later chapters.

CONCLUSION

Healthcare professionals require an ethical basis for their day-to-day work. The 'four-principle' model outlined above has its limitations and may not necessarily provide obvious answers, but it is a useful tool to identify and help in the analysis of ethical dilemmas.

From doing something seemingly straightforward such as performing a blood test to completing do-not-resuscitate orders, doctors are making ethical decisions – taking into account the patient's wishes (respecting his or her autonomy), weighing up the benefits against the possible harm of any medical action (beneficence and non-maleficence) and taking into consideration whether that action and its cost are fair overall (exercising justice).

The onus of such decision making no longer rests with the doctor alone. The media, the Internet and patient groups and advocates are providing the public with information about medicine and health on an unprecedented scale. This trend, together with the passing of the Human Rights Act, has brought the issue of patient autonomy to even greater prominence. In addition the rapid changes in modern medicine, ongoing research and increasing specialisation mean that ethical decision making requires the engagement not only of the patient and healthcare professionals but also of society at large.

REFERENCES

1 Beauchamp TL, Childress JF. *Principles of Biomedical Ethics*. 6th ed. New York: Oxford University Press; 2008.
2 Gillon R. Medical ethics: four principles plus attention to scope. *BMJ*. 1994; **309**: 184–8.
3 Hewson B. Why the Human Rights Act matters to doctors. *BMJ*. 2000; **321**: 780–1.
4 Gillon R. Ethics needs principles: four can encompass the rest and respect for autonomy should be first among equals'. *J Med Ethics*. 2003; **29**: 307–12.
5 Department of Health. *National Service Framework for Older People. Modern standards and service models*. London: Department of Health; 2001. Available at: www.dh.gov. uk/en/Publicationsandstatistics/Publications/PublicationsPolicyAndGuidance/ DH_4003066
6 Say RE, Thomson R. The importance of patient preferences in treatment decisions: challenges for doctors. *BMJ*. 2003; **327**: 542–5.
7 Coulter A. Patients' views of the good doctor. *BMJ*. 2002; **325**: 668–9.
8 Beauchamp TL, Childress JF. *Principles of Biomedical Ethics*. 5th ed. New York: Oxford University Press; 2001.
9 Garrett TM, Baillie HW, Garret RM. *Health Care: ethics, principles and problems*. 3rd ed. New Jersey: Prentice-Hall, Inc.; 1993.
10 Doyal L, Doyal L. Why active euthanasia and physician-assisted suicide should be legalised. *BMJ*. 2001; **323**: 1079–80.

FURTHER READING AND USEFUL WEBSITES

Beauchamp TL, Childress JF. *Principles of Biomedical Ethics*. 6th ed. New York: Oxford University Press; 2008.
Campbell AV, Gillett G, Jones G. *Medical Ethics*. 4th ed. Oxford: Oxford University Press; 2005.
Garrett TM, Ballie HW, Garrett RM. *Health Care: ethics, principles and problems*. New Jersey: Prentice-Hall, Inc.; 2001.
Journal of Medical Ethics. www.jme.bmj.com
UK Clinical Ethics Network. www.ethics-network.org.uk
www.gmc-uk.org.uk

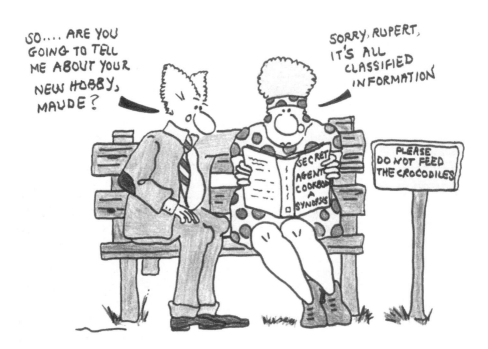

CHAPTER 2

Confidentiality

Catherine Harvey and Gurcharan S Rai

Confidentiality is one of the basic premises of medical practice and was enshrined in the Hippocratic oath:

> Whatever, in connection with my professional practice or not in connection with it, I see or hear, in the life of men, which ought not to be spoken of abroad, I will not divulge, as reckoning that all such should be kept secret.

This concept is now expressed in the professional codes of practice of healthcare professionals around the world. In the UK it is laid out in the General Medical Council's *Good Medical Practice*, which states that doctors have a duty to respect the privacy of patients and to protect the information given to them in confidence. Any information obtained in a professional capacity is subject to this. Consent should always be obtained before sharing this information with others, unless there are exceptional circumstances. Confidentiality is fundamental to a doctor–patient relationship, but doctors also have a duty of care to the community at large. This, coupled with the nature of information shared between doctors and their patients, can lead to conflicts of interest. When these occur and the question of breaching confidentiality arises, there must be clear ethical justification for doing so.

In addition to professional duties in maintaining confidentiality, there are legal requirements. Much of this has developed from case law in the UK. The Data Protection Act 1998 provides a framework outlining how information should be obtained, stored, used and shared. The Human Rights Act 1998 protects the privacy of individuals by Article 8 'The right to private and family life'.

THE IMPORTANCE OF CONFIDENTIALITY

The need for confidentiality is based on two principles:

1 the patient's right to privacy and autonomy
2 the preservation of a doctor–patient relationship that is based on mutual trust.

We choose carefully the information that we share with others. This information helps us to shape our identity – how we view ourselves, how we want others to see us and, to an extent, how they perceive us. Patients share sensitive information with their doctors about their physical, emotional, social and sexual health that they may not share with anyone else. The assumption of confidentiality means that they can do this without fear of embarrassment or disapproval. Without an implicit understanding that information will be kept private, patients may feel unable to talk to their doctor openly and frankly. Any barrier to open communication could make the already challenging task of appropriate investigation and therapy even more difficult. The fears of HIV and AIDS patients in the 1980s and 1990s illustrated the potential wide-ranging consequences of compromising confidentiality. There are implications for an individual's personal relationships, work and finance, as well as the possibility of discrimination.

In reality, the public's perception of what confidentiality means and the practice of modern medicine may differ significantly. This is partly because of the increasing numbers of people involved in providing medical care. It is particularly true when caring for older patients. Those involved can range from nursing staff and physiotherapists to carers and day-hospital receptionists. It is unlikely that patients are aware of the extent to which personal information is disseminated. There has also been an expansion in those who are not directly involved in patient care but who are involved in research and administration. Computerised records and the expansion of databases can also be seen to threaten our traditional idea of confidentiality.

Perhaps more pertinent for the majority of patients is how we deal with sensitive information on a busy ward or in a local general practice. Often life-changing discussions, such as breaking bad news, are conducted with just a curtain separating the patient from the outside world. Similarly, patients are openly discussed on a ward within hearing distance of other patients and relatives. Indiscretion is arguably the commonest form of breach of confidentiality. This may take the form of leaving notes open and unattended at a workstation or talking about patients to a colleague in a hospital canteen. Lapses can also occur when we are caring for older people who are very frail or with whom we find it difficult to communicate (e.g. due to deafness or dysarthria). We may find it simpler to talk to their next of kin. More detailed information is sometimes revealed to relatives and carers than to a patient, without having ensured the patient's consent.

SHARING INFORMATION WITH THE PATIENT'S CONSENT

Consent must be obtained before disclosing information to another party, unless there are exceptional circumstances. It is good practice to document this consent. Depending on the nature of the information being shared, this can be done formally with the patient's written consent or as a written record that verbal consent has been given. To give their consent, the patient should understand the nature and effects of the disclosure and have the capacity to make the decision.

It is essential that information is passed between health professionals to provide good healthcare. Clearly it is not always necessary to obtain explicit consent for this, provided that the patient has agreed to treatment or investigation. For instance, if a patient agrees to a specialist referral from their general practitioner (GP), then it is implied that they are happy for the GP to pass on details to the specialist. Patients expect health professionals to communicate in their best interests, and poor communication is a common source of frustration. However, difficulties can arise when patients and their doctors differ in their understanding of what information needs to be communicated and to whom. Only information that is relevant and required for optimum care should be disclosed, and it is the doctor's duty to ensure that the patient understands what information will be given.

If information is to be shared with others who are not involved in the healthcare of a patient, such as an employer or insurance company, then the patient's consent must be obtained. This should be done in writing prior to disclosure and should be limited to relevant information. It is the doctor's responsibility to ensure that the patient understands what information is shared and any adverse effects that such disclosures may have.

CASE 2.1

Mrs J is an active 87-year-old. She is admitted as an emergency case with dehydration due to vomiting. Investigation reveals a gastric malignancy that cannot be cured. On being told of the diagnosis, Mrs J is adamant that she does not want her family to be made aware of it. She says that she does not want her family treating her 'like a victim', and she wants to 'enjoy what is left of her life'. She has a large, caring extended family, who until this point have been fully informed of events, and who now want to know what is wrong with Mrs J.

Comment
Mrs J's wishes should be respected. It may help to discuss the impact of the decision with her. She may find it difficult to carry the burden of illness alone and find it hard to plan the rest of her time without the assistance of her family. At some stage in the course of her illness it is likely that they will discover the diagnosis

and will be hurt that they did not know about it sooner. Most importantly, dialogue should be kept open with Mrs J. Her views may change over time and she may value your support in discussions with her family at a later date.

SHARING INFORMATION WITHOUT CONSENT

In the UK, the principle of confidentiality is not considered absolute. It is not always possible to obtain consent to share personal information. This can occur in an emergency situation where it is not practical to do so, or when patients decide to withhold consent or do not have the capacity to give it. There are also circumstances when a doctor is required by law to disclose information. The General Medical Council offers guidance on situations when doctors may be justified in or required to disclose information that has been imparted to them in confidence. These can be summarised as follows:

1   when it is in the best interests of the patient or the public
2   when it is required by statute or law
3   for the purposes of medical research and education or public health.

Every attempt should be made to obtain consent. In the exceptional cases where it is not possible, the patient should be told of the decision to disclose information at the earliest opportunity. Only relevant information must be shared. Breaching confidentiality, even when justifiable, remains an infringement of the patient's rights, and doctors should be prepared to defend these decisions. It may be advisable to discuss the matter with a colleague or a professional body before arriving at such a decision.

In the patient's or public's best interests

It is sometimes necessary to divulge information without consent in the best interests of the public or a patient. Difficulties most often arise when a patient will not give consent but a doctor feels obliged to reveal information. In such a situation the potential benefits of making a disclosure need to be carefully weighed against the harm caused to the patient and the loss of faith in the medical profession for that patient and for others. Attempts should always be made to persuade the patient to share information voluntarily or to give their consent to this. It might be helpful to ask the patient hypothetically what they would do if they were in the doctor's position. For patients who are unable to give consent because they lack capacity to do so, decisions must be made in accordance with Mental Capacity Act 2005.

CASE 2.2

Mr D has been diagnosed with early dementia. He looks after his wife, who is physically impaired following a stroke. He tells you that he relies on his car to do the shopping and to take his wife out on trips that contribute greatly to their quality of life. You are concerned that Mr D may no longer be safe behind the wheel. You tell him he must contact the Driver and Vehicle Licensing Authority (DVLA) and tell them of his diagnosis. He insists that he will not do this because he must be allowed to continue driving. You judge that he has capacity to make this decision.

Comment

The DVLA have clear requirements. Dementia is one of the diagnoses they must be informed of. If Mr D is not deemed safe to drive, there is a risk to both him and his wife and also to the public. He is legally obliged to tell the DVLA of his diagnosis. His doctor should tell him this and that the DVLA will not automatically revoke his license on the basis of the diagnosis alone. If he still refuses to inform the DVLA, then it is the duty of his doctor to inform them. Mr D should be made aware of this.

Decisions where there is conflict between the rights of known individuals and of others are most challenging when the degree of harm and the probability of harm are hard to quantify. A doctor's duty to the public may prevail if a disclosure may assist in the prevention, detection or prosecution of serious crime. If there is a risk of death or serious harm, then the doctor is required to disclose information. Again, only relevant information should be shared and it should not be used for other purposes.

CASE 2.3

Mr W is a 75-year-old who has been admitted with a chest infection. He is thin and unkempt and has a number of bruises on his arms and chest. He lives with his son and relies on him for help with getting washed and dressed, to prepare meals and do his cleaning and shopping. When his son has visited the ward, he has smelt of alcohol. Nurses raise the possibility of abuse and think that you should inform social services or the police. Mr W will not discuss the matter and says that he wants to go home to his son.

Comment

Elder abuse can take the form of physical, emotional, sexual, financial abuse or neglect. There are no specific laws in the UK to protect the elderly from these. They are subject to the same laws as other, younger adults. Mr W is dependent on a close family member who may or may not be guilty of neglect or abuse. However, he remains a competent adult capable of making his own decisions and has the right to determine what information he shares with others. It would be wise to suggest supportive measures for Mr W and his son. The introduction of a care package may help to reduce stress on the family. It will provide a point of contact with external services, should he need assistance. Any decision to breach confidentiality in such an instance needs to take into account the risk of serious harm to the individual or others, the vulnerability of the individual and the nature and impact of abuse. If Mr W lacked capacity to make these judgements, then further action would be needed to safeguard him. Institutions involved in the care of vulnerable adults should have a policy outlining the process which should be undertaken when abuse is suspected.

Legal process

In a court of law, a judge can order the disclosure of information. A doctor can object if he or she believes that the information is irrelevant but the decision falls to the judge.

Information should not be given to either lawyers or police without consent. The only exception to this is where failure to disclose information would put people at risk of serious harm. The definition of 'serious crime' or 'harm' is a grey area but the National Health Service (NHS) code of practice suggests it includes rape, murder, manslaughter, neglect and assault. Information must also be disclosed if there is a statutory obligation to do so – for example, in the notification of certain infectious diseases or in cases of substance misuse.

The Data Protection Act 1998 and Access to Health Records Act 1990 give health professionals the right not to disclose information if they believe that disclosure is likely to cause serious harm to the physical or mental health of the patient or of any other person.

Medical research, education and public health

Information obtained in clinical practice is used for other purposes, including medical research, education and audit. These do not directly benefit an individual patient but are of use to society as a whole (e.g. in improving patient safety or in health planning). While sharing much of this kind of information poses little threat to an individual, it has still been imparted in confidence, and the use and protection of such data has been controversial. In broad terms: information should only be given to those who are also bound by a duty of confidentiality; consent should be sought to share information; and data should be anonymous. Local research ethics committees ensure that research proposals are robust and take confidentiality into account. Each health organisation also has a Caldicott Guardian. Their role is to protect the confidentiality of information and to ensure lawful and ethical information sharing. The Health and Social Care Act 2001 authorises the Secretary of State to allow patient-identifiable information to be shared without consent when it is in the wider public interest in improving medical care (e.g. cancer registries).

CASE 2.4

Mrs B's family comes to visit her in hospital. They are incensed to find a medical student reading their mother's notes at the nurse's desk.

Comment
The value of confidentiality needs to be impressed upon medical students and other trainee health professionals from an early stage of their training. Most patients recognise the importance of medical education and are keen to assist in it. It can be argued that the medical student in this case should have obtained consent to read the notes, as they would have done before taking a history from the patient or carrying out a physical examination.

More and more data are being stored on information technology systems. Electronic health records are increasingly available. The NHS is developing the Patient Care Record containing a summary of a patient's health details. This will allow information to be shared between healthcare providers such as GPs and hospital trusts. Publicity surrounding the loss of information by other public bodies has led to concern about how information is stored and protected and how it can be accessed.

The Data Protection Act 1998 safeguards information whether it is held in paper form, electronically on computer or in another medium such as pictures. On a day-to-day basis, it is important that users take the same care with computer records as they would with medical notes. This means not leaving screens unattended, remembering to log off and not sharing passwords.

RELEASE OF INFORMATION AFTER DEATH

CASE 2.5

The nephew of an 89-year-old Greek patient who had attended an outpatient department for investigations and management of diabetes and abnormal liver function tests a year earlier, makes an appointment to see the consultant. At the meeting, he informs the consultant that his aunt died six months ago. Before her death, her brother persuaded her sign a Will while she was ill in hospital. The

Will left all of her estate to her brother. The nephew suspects that this Will does not represent the wishes of his aunt, for it is written in English and her English was poor. He asks for copies of medical records which state that his aunt could not communicate in English and that at each outpatient visit an interpreter was required.

Comment
Good communication with bereaved families is very important. However, even after a patient has died a doctor still has a duty of confidentiality. Doctors should not disclose any information if the patient has requested non-disclosure and this is documented in the medical records. While records for living patients are protected by the Data Protection Act, the records of deceased patients are governed by the Access to Medical Records Act 1990. The deceased patient's personal representative has the right to access their medical records. This is the executor of their Will and not necessarily their next of kin. Others who have a claim arising out of a patient's death may also have access to records. In this instance, it is advisable to seek legal advice.

ACCESS TO MEDICAL REPORTS

Medical reports commonly prepared by practitioners for employment and insurance purposes are based on confidential information provided by an individual to the doctor. Under the Access to Medical Reports Act 1988, the patient has a right to inspect or be supplied with a copy of their medical reports. However, a report prepared by an independent practitioner who has not treated the person and who has never been involved in his or her care is not covered by the Medical Reports Act 1988 or the Data Protection Act 1998.

KEY POINTS

- Doctors have a duty to keep confidential any information that is learned in a professional capacity.
- The Data Protection Act 1998 and the Human Rights Act 1998 (the right to freedom) confirm a responsibility to prevent disclosure of information that has been imparted in confidence.
- Breaches of confidentiality are most often unintentional or careless (e.g. discussing a patient with a colleague in a lift, leaving notes or computer records unattended on a ward, talking to relatives without a patient's consent).
- Consent must be obtained to share information unless there are exceptional circumstances. This may be in the public's or in a patient's best interests, when required to by law or for the purposes of medical research.

- Careful consideration must be given to breaching confidentiality in these circumstances. Doctors must be prepared to justify these. If in doubt, seek legal advice.
- In broad terms, for the purposes of medical research, education and public health, information should only be given to those who are bound by a duty of confidentiality, consent should be sought to share information and data should be anonymous.
- The duty of confidentiality persists after the death of a patient and medical records should only be shared with their personal representative.

FURTHER READING

Action on Elder Abuse. *Safeguarding Adults: a National Framework of Standards for good practice and outcomes in adult protection work*. London: AEA; 2005. Available at: www. elderabuse.org.uk/Useful%20downloads/ADSS/SAFEGUARDING%20ADULTS.pdf

Beauchamp TL, Childress JF. Professional–patient relationships. In: *Principles of Biomedical Ethics*. 5th ed. Oxford: Oxford University Press; 2001.

Bourke J, Wessely S. Confidentiality. *BMJ*. 2008; **336**: 888–91.

British Medical Association. *Confidentiality and Disclosure of Health Information* [tool kit]. London: British Medical Association; 2008.

General Medical Council. *Confidentiality: protecting and providing information*. London: GMC; 2004. Available at: www.gmc-uk.org/guidance/current/library/confidentiality. asp (accessed 14 April 2009).

Mason JK, Laurie GT. Medical confidentiality. In: JK Mason, GT Laurie, editors. *Mason & McCall Smith's Law and Medical Ethics*. 7th ed. Oxford: Oxford University Press; 2006.

NHS Code of Practice: *Confidentiality*. London: DoH; 2005. Available at: www.dh.gov. uk/en/Publicationsandstatistics/Publications/PublicationsPolicyAndGuidance/DH_4069253 (accessed 14 April 2009).

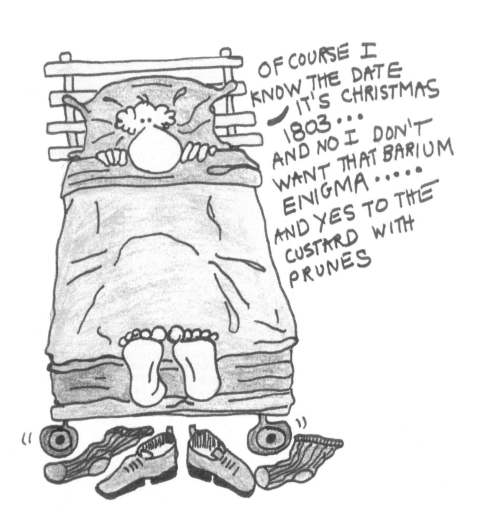

CHAPTER 3

Informed consent

Sally Briggs and Martin J Vernon

INTRODUCTION

The last two decades have seen positive and sustained movement towards person-centred care for older people.[1,2] Patient choice is fundamental to good medical practice.[3] Who would contemplate forcing treatment on an individual against their wishes or without seeking their views? Consent pervades all aspects of clinical work, and yet it often remains nothing more than a mundane procedure which begins and ends with the signing of a consent form. In many situations consent passes without difficulty, sometimes even unnoticed by the parties concerned. However, when the process breaks down, health workers are often left wondering how best to proceed. In these circumstances an understanding of the underlying professional, moral and legal issues can help to resolve the dilemmas which ensue.

Healthcare for older people is particularly fraught with problems concerning consent. Physical and mental impairments may hinder the normal dialogue which occurs between doctor and patient, thereby obstructing the usual consent process. At worst, this leads to a complete failure of the process, either because the patient is unable or unwilling to provide consent, or because the doctor is unable or unwilling to seek consent. The following familiar case examples illustrate these problems.

CASE 3.1 A PATIENT UNABLE TO PROVIDE CONSENT

Dr Smith wishes to obtain a sample of blood from her patient, Harry, who sufferers from dementia and is profoundly confused. He spends much of his day staring out of a window and rarely talks. The doctor tries to explain her intentions to Harry, but he cries out loudly and pulls away when she lifts his arm and tries to insert the needle.

CASE 3.2 A PATIENT UNWILLING TO PROVIDE CONSENT

Dr Smith wishes to obtain a sample of blood from her patient, Sarah, who is awaiting surgery for a fractured neck of femur. The doctor tries to explain her intentions, but Sarah shrugs and says that at her time of life she does not want to be 'pulled about' and is much happier being left alone, 'whatever the consequences'.

CASE 3.3 A DOCTOR UNABLE TO SEEK CONSENT

Dr Smith wishes to obtain a sample of blood from her patient, Pauline, who has severely impaired hearing. The doctor tries to explain her intentions to Pauline, who smiles but does not otherwise respond. Dr Smith is left feeling uncertain as to how much has been understood.

CASE 3.4 A DOCTOR UNWILLING TO SEEK CONSENT

Dr Smith wishes to obtain a sample of blood from her patient, Michael, who has suffered a stroke and has expressive dysphasia. The doctor tries to explain her intentions to Michael, who attempts to respond but struggles to get the words out. Dr Smith listens to him struggling for a few minutes, but is in a hurry and decides to proceed before Michael has finished trying to express himself. He becomes tearful during the procedure, and the doctor later worries about the correctness of her actions.

By presenting a structured approach to the consent process, this chapter seeks to provide assistance in resolving dilemmas which are commonly encountered in delivering healthcare to older people. While it is tempting to resort to legal frameworks when deciding right from wrong, there are many situations where the law is unhelpful or even silent. A more pragmatic approach is to consider the moral basis of the consent process, and to work from first principles towards a solution which is consistent with the law, rather than dictated by it.

THE BASIS OF CONSENT
Professional duties
It is helpful to look at the values which underlie the duties of health professionals. The various strands of professional practice on which the notion of consent is based are readily discernible in a variety of professional mandates.

For example, in the Hippocratic oath attention is drawn to the importance of acting only for a patient's benefit, and avoiding doing them harm:

> I will prescribe regimen for the good of my patients according to my ability and judgement and never do harm to anyone . . . In every house where I come I will enter only for the good of my patients, keeping myself far from all intentional ill-doing.[4]

The General Medical Council, in setting out the duties of a doctor, has focused on the importance of consent in maintaining trust:

> Patients must be able to trust doctors with their lives and health. To justify that trust you must:
> ➤ make the care of your patient your first concern
> ➤ treat patients as individuals and respect their dignity
> ➤ listen to patients and respond to their concerns and preferences
> ➤ give patients the information they want or need in a way they can understand
> ➤ respect patients' right to reach decisions with you about their treatment and care
> ➤ be honest and open and act with integrity.[3]

The moral basis of consent

Although specifically directed towards doctors, intuitively these declarations are more generally applicable. On closer inspection, three common themes emerge:
➤ avoidance of doing intentional harm
➤ promotion of benefit and well-being
➤ respect for the wishes and desires of the individual.

Each of these relates to a particular moral principle, and it is helpful to briefly consider each of them in turn.

Non-maleficence

This principle creates an obligation not to do intentional harm to others, and there are a number of ways of achieving this. Most obviously we should try not to do things which cause harm, but we may also be obliged to stop or prevent processes which are causing harm to an individual. It is helpful to decide what we mean by 'harm' in this situation. Although we ordinarily think of harm as meaning physical or psychological injury, there are other ways in which the interests of an individual may be damaged.

Returning to Dr Smith and her blood samples, we might conclude that Harry has been physically harmed when he cries out on being touched, but Michael's tearfulness also suggests harm, despite his showing no resistance to the procedure. This may be more than the pain of having blood taken, and may equally well relate to his thwarted attempts to express a view. In Sarah's case, the patient has expressed clearly that she does not want a blood test and that she is best left alone. Ignoring her wishes would both undermine her interests in being left alone and damage the trust that she maintains with her carers. Such action may thus harm the integrity of future decision making.

Beneficence

This principle requires us to act so as to contribute to the welfare of individuals, and it is closely allied to non-maleficence. We might choose to do this by actively providing benefit for a person, or by not restricting opportunities for benefit. Alternatively, we may choose to balance the benefits and drawbacks of a situation in order to arrive at the best outcome.

Dr Smith's cases provide some illustration of this principle. Her intention in obtaining the blood samples is presumably to derive information which will contribute to the welfare of her patients. By having open discussions with the patients, she has sought to avoid restricting their opportunities. If the patient has expressed a view, at least it can be taken into account. By balancing the benefits and drawbacks for her patient, the doctor may be better placed to arrive at a decision on how to proceed. Such a calculation would depend on factors such as the magnitude of benefit to be derived from doing the test, and the amount of harm done by overriding any objections that the patient might have.

Respect for autonomy

Respect for the wishes of an individual is perhaps at the root of morally robust consent. The concept of autonomy, although difficult to grasp, comprises elements of freedom from interference and capacity for action. In deciding whether to be influenced by an individual's views, it is useful to consider whether they are or can be autonomous. One view is that someone is autonomous if they:
➤ have plans free from interference by others
➤ have thought about these plans critically
➤ are free to carry out their plans.

Thinking about Dr Smith's patients, it could be argued that Harry's dementia prevents him from being autonomous. He does not appear to have the mental capacity to think about any plans. If he does have plans, his impairment is likely to constrain him in their execution. It could be argued that overriding his refusal does not conflict with the principle of respect for autonomy, since he is not autonomous. Sarah, on the other hand, clearly wants to be left alone, 'whatever the consequences', indicating that she has at least considered that there may be consequences to her refusing the test. Adherents to the principle of respect for autonomy would be unable to justify overriding her refusal, unless other grounds for questioning her autonomy could be found.

Where there is sufficient evidence that an individual is autonomous, it is difficult to justify proceeding in the face of a clear refusal. However, where the evidence to establish autonomy is lacking, decisions about an individual's autonomy can be difficult. In this situation it is useful to consider instead the notion of an *autonomous choice*.[5] What matters here is whether the individual has *actually* made a free decision about their care, rather than whether they are capable of being autonomous. Dr Smith and her patients provide a useful illustration of this. Although Harry's dementia deprives him of autonomous status, he has nevertheless clearly indicated that he does not want a needle stuck in his arm. Whatever the reason for this response, it is a powerful demonstration that, despite his dementia, he can still state a preference to be left alone.

PROBLEMS WITH RESPECT FOR AUTONOMY

Is there an over-reliance on the principle of respect for autonomy? While a patient retains autonomy we should respect their choices, whatever the outcome and so long as others are not harmed as a consequence. When autonomy is absent, the patient's views are no longer central to decision making. In a way, this lets health workers off the moral hook. They need no longer worry about a patient who is choosing 'unwisely', because that choice does not demand respect. Instead, the views of others decide what should happen. The practice of allowing health workers to determine whether an individual is autonomous could effectively displace the balance of power in decision making away from the patient. Strict adherence to the principle of respect for autonomy could paradoxically lead to higher levels of paternalism if health workers are reluctant to grant their patients autonomous status.

The problem arises from the view that autonomy is either present or absent. The solution lies with willingness to permit 'partial autonomy' and to treat patients as people. The right to determine what should happen to oneself could therefore be granted on either ability to choose or preservation of self (personhood).

Partial autonomy

Even in a 'free' society there are rules which restrict action and choice, so that no adult is completely autonomous. It is simply unrealistic to require a patient to have full autonomy before respecting their choices. However, surely a patient who is able to order and choose between their various desires (e.g. to eat, mobilise, or be free from pain) is deserving of respect? Arguably only a patient who exhibits no such ability should be excluded from the consent process.

Personhood

Loss of this characteristic may indeed justify excluding the patient from a decision about their healthcare. However, many individuals without full autonomy will continue to be recognised as persons. The presence of actions that display purpose, awareness and intent together with a recognition of 'self' by external observers should prompt respect for preservation of personhood. Despite his dementia, Harry still presents himself as a person to his carers. Arguably the doctor should respect his choice because he remains a person despite being unable to demonstrate that he is an autonomous individual.

THE ANATOMY OF CONSENT

Consent in clinical practice may assume a variety of guises, from an explicit, fully informed dialogue to a tacit, implied authorisation. It is also important to remember that a significant aspect of the consent process is to provide choice for the patient, and that the outcome of that process may be either acceptance or refusal of an intervention. It is certainly not the purpose of the consent process to secure acceptance at all costs.

A further point to be noted is that the consent is an authorisation or refusal of an intervention offered to a particular individual, and unjustified attempts to exclude that individual from the process are likely to conflict with the principles of non-maleficence, beneficence and respect for autonomy. In other words, obtaining consent (or refusal) from any individual other than the one to whom the intervention directly relates must be clearly justified both morally and by applicable legal frameworks.

To ensure the validity of the consent process, it is widely agreed that a number of elements are essential:
➤ capacity
➤ information
➤ voluntariness.

Capacity

The notions of capacity and autonomy are closely related, and it has been demonstrated that decisions about whether an individual is autonomous can be troublesome, particularly where evidence in favour of autonomy is lacking. Recent changes in English law have sought to clarify matters in respect of adults. The Mental Capacity Act 2005[6] is underpinned by five key principles:
1 an adult is presumed to have capacity unless proven otherwise
2 individuals should be supported as far as possible to make their own decisions
3 an unwise decision does not mean that an individual lacks capacity
4 a decision made for someone lacking capacity must be done in their best interests

5 anything done for someone lacking capacity must be the option that least
   restricts their basic rights and freedoms.

For the purposes of the Act, a person lacks capacity in relation to a matter if at
the material time they are unable to make a decision for themselves because
of an impairment or disturbance in the functioning of the mind or brain. This
means that a person lacks capacity if:
➤ they have an impairment or disturbance that affects the way their mind or
   brain works, and
➤ the impairment or disturbance means that they are unable to make a
   specific decision at the time it needs to be made.[6]

For legal purposes, capacity is either present or absent, but a decision about the
capacity of an individual will depend on the specific circumstances of the consent situation. For example, where an intervention carries little risk and great
benefit to the individual, there maybe little information for the individual to
comprehend and process, and the decision may not be difficult to make. In this
situation, a patient with significant impairment may nevertheless be judged to
have capacity to make the decision. Where the risks and benefits of a procedure
are more finely balanced, the complexity of information necessary to arrive at
a decision may increase, so that even unimpaired patients may have difficulty
reaching the standard of capacity required to make the decision.
     Capacity can be assessed by any suitably trained healthcare professional
and considers an individual's ability to understand the relevant information
provided, retain the information and use it to make a decision. They must then
have the ability to communicate their decision. If there is a temporary impairment of cognition (e.g. during a delirium), it must be considered whether a
particular decision can wait.

Information

The information provided can influence decisions about capacity, but it can
also influence the consent process in other ways. The notion of fully informed
consent is particularly problematic. How much information does a patient actually require to make the decision? The patient may be at a distinct disadvantage
if the professional decides to withhold certain facts. The reasons for doing so
may be perfectly valid. For instance, if the information is considered harmful
to the patient (so-called therapeutic privilege), or the professional simply does
not know the facts.
     In addition to problems of disclosure, consent may be obstructed by prob-
lems of understanding. The demonstration of understanding can be difficult and
requires considerable experience. Dr Smith's discussion with Sarah illustrates
the point well. She expresses the view that at her age she does not want to be

treated, but this may be based on the mistaken belief that nothing can be done for older people with fractured hips. Although competent, she has misunderstood the purpose of the intervention because of a defect in the information she has been given.

A useful approach to problems of information is to address the needs of the individual, and it is important to check with the patient that they have enough information to make a decision. Where understanding is in question, it may be prudent to wait (if the urgency for the intervention is not great) until understanding is sufficient. This may mean spending considerably more time than is usual in ensuring that information has been properly communicated and understood.

Voluntariness

Healthcare decisions should be free from undue influence, and here it is helpful to refer again to the principle of respect for autonomy. The patient may be influenced by the views of the health worker, while physical or mental impairments may also restrict freedom in decision making. It should also be remembered that patient freedom may be viewed in a positive sense of providing all available opportunities, or in a negative sense of not restricting opportunity.

Let us return to the case of Michael. His expressive dysphasia considerably limited his powers of expression, and in such situations it may be easier for the patient to nod an agreement than to try to explain their reasons for refusal of a procedure. Similar arguments could be mounted for Pauline, whose profound sensory impairments limit her freedom of expression. In this sense, neither patient could be said to be truly free to make decisions.

Where a patient is either unwilling or unable to provide consent, it is helpful to consider whether the individual is free from adverse influence. Such influence may be either intrinsic as a consequence of their impairments, or extrinsic as a result of coercion by others. An effort should be made to address these issues and to reduce their impact on decision making, thereby improving the validity of the consent process.

THE FORM OF CONSENT

When an intervention such as a surgical procedure is perceived to be of sufficient importance, the ritual of making the consent explicit may involve written documentation or a structured conversation with the patient. Where the intervention is more 'trivial', the patient's agreement may be assumed and the issue of consent then becomes tacit or implied. In the latter situation it is easy to forget about the need for consent altogether.

Making the consent process explicit in all clinical encounters could rapidly undermine the smooth and efficient administration of healthcare, to the ultimate detriment of the patient. For example, it would be ludicrous to expect written documentation of agreement for each of the tasks entailed in day-to-day care. Nevertheless, the absence of explicit consent does not equate to the absence of need for consent, and it must be remembered that consent is an issue whenever a medical intervention is contemplated.

WHEN THERE IS NO VALID CONSENT

Despite the ubiquitous nature of consent, there will be many situations in the practice of elderly care where there is simply no valid consent or refusal to be obtained. It will be clear that acceptance of this state of affairs should not be taken lightly, since due consideration must be given to factors which may be blighting the consent process. In addition, the moral validity of a consent process may be influenced by the values of health workers themselves, depending, for example, upon their particular conception of respect for autonomy or non-maleficence.

The Mental Capacity Act has for the first time in England and Wales enabled individuals to appoint a lasting power of attorney (LPA) to make decisions about welfare, property and affairs on their behalf should they lose capacity. If no LPA has been appointed, then decisions made must be in a person's best interests.

Best interests

Best interests specifically does not apply where: 1) a competent individual has already made an explicit advance refusal of the healthcare intervention being proposed, and 2) in some instances relating to research. All interested parties should meet to try and decide what the person would have wished had they had capacity to make their own decisions. The Mental Capacity Act helpfully provides a checklist to ensure that all relevant issues have been considered[6]:

➤ determining best interests cannot be simply based on age, appearance, condition or behaviour.
➤ all relevant circumstances should be considered.
➤ every effort should be made to encourage and enable the person who lacks capacity to take part in the decision.
➤ if there is a chance that capacity will be regained, consider putting off the decision until this occurs.
➤ particular caution must be applied to decisions about life-sustaining treatment
➤ the person's past and present wishes and feelings, beliefs and values should be taken into account
➤ the views of others close to the individual should be considered.

As much background as possible about the person should be obtained, and any relatives or close contacts should be included in the process. If a person has no family or friends to advocate on their behalf, then an independent mental capacity advocate (IMCA) may be arranged to support the decision-making process. The team must weigh the interests that an individual might have in receiving an intervention compared with those they might have in not receiving it. Such a calculation might involve weighing the pain and suffering likely to be caused against the possible benefits of having the procedure. This will in turn depend on the nature of the procedure. For example, Dr Smith is likely to cause Harry great distress by persisting in taking blood, but the balance of interests in having the test will shift according to the reason for taking the blood. If the test is for a research project, the outcome of which is unlikely to benefit Harry, then it is unlikely to be in his best interests. However, if it is to cross-match blood for a much-needed transfusion, the balance of interests shifts the other way. Individual professionals' values should not be allowed to influence the decision-making process.

CONSENT TO RESEARCH

The morality of the consent process with regard to research involving older people is essentially no different from that of other healthcare interventions. Nevertheless, the emergence of research ethics committees as 'gatekeepers' in the conduct of research involving vulnerable people has ensured that the consent process for research is generally more explicit and complete than in other aspects of clinical practice.

An area of particular difficulty relates to research involving patients for whom there is no valid consent or refusal (e.g. those with severe dementia). Surrogate decision making in this context is more problematic, since the benefits to the patient may be less obvious, unknown or even non-existent. It is unlikely that interests will weigh strongly in favour of conducting the research. It is equally unlikely that an advance directive will have anticipated the nature of future research in sufficiently specific detail to permit authorisation.

Once again, strict adherence to the principle of respect for autonomy is problematic. As a result of excluding from research those patients who are unable to consent, both their condition and its treatment remain less well understood. Arguably this is just as morally unacceptable as engaging in experimentation on vulnerable adults without seeking their agreement. A way forward is to permit decisions by adults who have partial autonomy or who retain the characteristics of personhood. In practice, this might involve respecting the patient's assent to participate in research in the absence of obvious refusal. However, it is likely that research ethics committees will remain reluctant to authorise such an approach because of the potential for abuse.

KEY POINTS

- Freely given consent to healthcare is a moral and legal imperative.
- For older people, problems may arise because a patient is unwilling or unable to provide consent, or because the carer is unwilling or unable to seek consent.
- An understanding of the moral basis of consent will help to provide solutions to consent problems which are consistent with the law.
- The moral basis of consent is derived from the principles of non-maleficence, beneficence and respect for autonomy.
- Reliance on respect for autonomy may lead to paternalism by excluding individuals who can still choose despite cognitive impairment.
- A morally and legally valid consent requires the patient to be competent, informed and voluntary.
- Consent may be explicit or tacit, but is relevant to all healthcare interventions.
- When an adult cannot provide valid consent, healthcare decisions may be justified on the basis of best interests or in line with advance directives for healthcare.

REFERENCES

1 Department of Health. *National Service Framework for Older People: modern standards and service models.* London: Department of Health; 2001. Available at: www.dh.gov. uk/en/Publicationsandstatistics/Publications/PublicationsPolicyAndGuidance/ DH_4003066
2 British Geriatrics Society. www.bgs.org.uk
3 General Medical Council. www.gmc-uk.org
4 Mason JK, Laurie GT, editors. *Mason and McCall Smith's Law and Medical Ethics.* 7th ed. Oxford: Oxford University Press; 2006.
5 Beauchamp TL, Childress JF. *Principles of Biomedical Ethics.* 6th ed. New York: Oxford University Press; 2008.
6 Department of Health. *Mental Capacity Act 2005.* London: Department of Health; 2005. Available at: www.justice.gov.uk

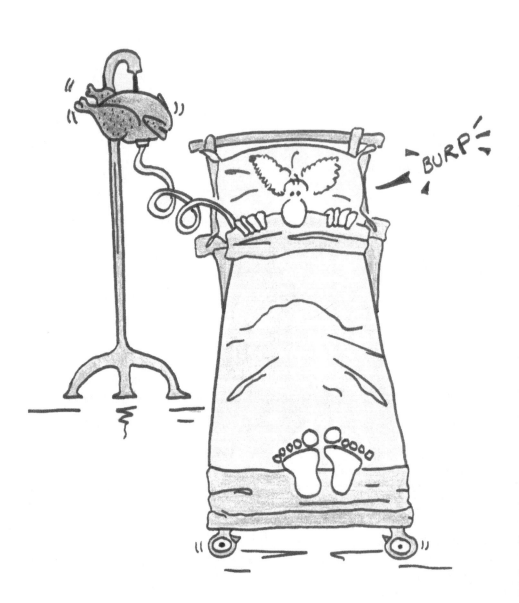

CHAPTER 4

Decisions on life-sustaining therapy: nutrition and fluid

Sally Briggs and Martin J Vernon

INTRODUCTION

The continued receipt of food and water is fundamental to life, and to deny an individual these essential substrates seems morally indefensible. One only need conjure up media images of people starving as a result of environmental or man-made catastrophe to be reminded of the appalling consequences of malnutrition. The issues surrounding nutrition and hydration in the care of older people are perhaps less obvious, although no less important. In recent years there has been increasing media attention with headlines claiming that hospitals and doctors are starving older people to death. While raising public awareness, there is nonetheless a danger of over-simplification and populism when celebrity chefs take on the issue for the purpose of good television. In England, the Department of Health has responded to the issue by producing an action plan[1] to improve nutritional care which focuses on older people and highlights the importance of issues such as screening, protected mealtimes and education of staff throughout healthcare settings.

Older people are at risk of malnutrition for a variety of reasons, particularly socio-economic deprivation and a higher prevalence of physical and cognitive impairments than younger adults. In one of the very few UK hospital studies, up to 40% of acute admissions to elderly care wards were judged to be under-nourished, with one in five severely so. In comparison, only one in 12 general medical and one in 100 general surgical admissions were judged to be severely undernourished.[2] Interestingly, the same study revealed that the majority of those who were undernourished on admission became more so during their hospital stay, indicating that nutrition should be high on the management agenda for ill older people. Research[3,4,5] has suggested that malnutrition is associated with increased mortality, rate of complications, length of stay and readmission rates. It is not an issue that can be ignored.

When deciding whether or not to feed an older patient who is unable to take sufficient nutrition orally, three main strands of argument commonly emerge:

1 are there any scientific principles which may support a particular course of action?
2 what is the technical feasibility of pursuing that course?
3 what are the moral principles underlying those actions?

Scientific principles

Is there any evidence that feeding the patient will do some good? Malnutrition affects many organ systems, leading to (among other things) impairments of central nervous, cardiorespiratory and immune function, cognition and tissue repair.[6] Patients who are already challenged by pathological changes in one or more of these systems are more likely to suffer the consequences of malnutrition, leading to increased healthcare costs, morbidity and mortality. The inference of this is that supplemental nutrition may reduce the impact of some or all of these effects, speeding recovery and reducing the length of hospital stay for patients following an acute illness. This notion has been confirmed in some studies of older patients undergoing rehabilitation.[6]

Yet malnutrition may result from dementia or progressive neurological impairment, where the desire or ability to eat has been lost. Ought we to consider artificial nutrition and hydration (ANH) to maximise the chances of survival and reduce discomfort? Should we offer this on the grounds of palliation to all patients regardless of diagnosis or prognosis? Or are there situations where there is no benefit and only harm as a consequence of ANH?

Reasons for considering ANH in older patients range from attempts to avoid aspiration pneumonia, pressure ulcers or disability to the prevention or delay of death. However, there is mounting evidence that in some circumstances ANH may not offer the benefits intended.[7] Studies suggest that ANH is often ineffective in achieving these objectives while continuing to expose patients to potential harm.[8]

On the other hand, is there any evidence that not feeding a given patient is necessarily harmful? Can the absence of nutrition be beneficial in certain circumstances? For example, the feeding of dying patients can lead to unwanted or potentially harmful effects, such as increased hunger, thirst, nausea and agitation, while in some circumstances removal of hydration may increase patient comfort. Contrast this with a 30-day mortality rate in excess of 20% following percutaneous feeding gastrostomy placement.[9]

When contemplating ANH, it is therefore important first to consider the alternative options. For patients with advanced dementia who are experiencing

swallowing difficulties, stopping anti-cholinergic medication, sedatives, neu-
roleptics or non-steroidal anti-inflammatory drugs may be sufficient to improve
their nutritional intake. Any reversible illnesses such as sepsis or depression
should be treated. Missing or ill-fitting dentures should be remedied! Other
strategies include the education of care staff in how to safely feed patients at
risk, the use of strong flavours and finger foods, or a change in the frequency
and size of meals. With such measures, survival rates with or without ANH may
be no different.[10]

Technical feasibility

Where nutritional support may be beneficial but oral feeding is impossible,
what are the alternative means of accomplishing feeding? There is now a range
of options at our disposal, including intravenous (IV), nasogastric (NG), percutaneous endoscopic gastrostomy (PEG), radiographically inserted gastrostomy
(RIG) or peri-oral image-guided gastrostomy (PIG). However, in common with
many other healthcare interventions, the availability of these techniques does
not resolve the problem of whether it is right to employ this technology for a
particular patient.

Moral principles

Clarifying the scientific evidence, together with an understanding of what is possible, will focus the decision-making process. Although helpful, this approach
alone may not yield a morally robust solution to a clinical dilemma. Where
there is no evidence of benefit from an intervention, or evidence that it might
do great harm, there may be little debate. Often, however, the evidence supports
several courses of action to which there are no particular technical barriers. A
decision must then be made as to the right course of action in each individual
situation.

   With regard to decisions about nutrition for older patients, two morally
important questions commonly arise:
1 should we feed (and/or hydrate) this person?
2 should we stop feeding (and/or hydrating) this person?

This chapter seeks to develop a framework for addressing these questions, and
assumes that there is at least some scientific evidence in favour of the courses of
action available, and that such actions are at least technically possible.

   In practice, nutrition and hydration are usually provided simultaneously,
and the discussion will assume this to be the case. Although some clinical
situations require decisions solely about hydration, it is recommended that
dilemmas relating to hydration are approached in the same way as those concerning nutrition.

MEDICAL TREATMENT OR BASIC CARE?

In developing a morally robust solution to the dilemma of whether or not to feed an older patient, it is necessary to consider first whether nutritional support constitutes medical therapy or basic humane care. Those who support the view that it is medical therapy have invoked the moral imperatives driving good professional practice to decide on the appropriateness of proposed treatment.[11,12] Those who adhere to the view that food is a basic necessity of life, irrespective of how it is given, have developed arguments along more humanitarian lines, free from the encumbrances of professional codes of practice.

It is interesting to note that the procedural nature of supplemental nutrition has a significant impact on its categorisation, and therefore on the moral arguments which surround its application. Consider the following clinical scenario.

CASE 4.1

Jodie has been admitted to hospital with pneumonia. At the time of admission, she is judged to be malnourished. She is given 'three square meals' of hospital food per day, but continues to lose weight. She is reviewed by a dietitian, who recommends supplementation and gives her cartons of liquid nutrients which she enjoys drinking. One week after admission she suffers a stroke and is unable to swallow. Nasogastric feeding is commenced and she makes good progress with rehabilitation. Unfortunately, one month later she is diagnosed with a carcinoma of the large bowel which is threatening to obstruct. The surgical team is prepared to operate, but first requests intravenous feeding to optimise her chances of recovery from the surgery.

At what point does the nutritional support which Jodie requires constitute medical therapy? 'Three square meals' does not appear to constitute medical therapy, since no specific procedure is involved and she is free to eat normally. At first glance, it would appear that her meals assume the moral status of a basic necessity of life. Nevertheless, one could present an alternative view. She is now in a medical environment which is in itself therapeutic. It is not merely the antibiotics she receives for her pneumonia which will help to restore her health, but the attentions and care of a full multi-disciplinary team including nurses, therapists, dietitian and doctors. The food she is receiving is part of this therapeutic process, and as such is subject to the same level of supervision and monitoring as other unarguably therapeutic aspects of her care.

Further support for this view arises when it becomes necessary for a nurse or other skilled professional to supervise feeding, perhaps because the patient is at risk of aspiration. Although the patient may be consuming normal food, the process of eating can be achieved safely only with skilled intervention.

Similar arguments could be presented for the liquid nutrients that Jodie is given. Such drinks are readily available outside the medical environment and could simply be viewed as a 'health food'. Alternatively, they could assume the status of a treatment by assisting the management of her medical conditions which have been worsened as a result of malnutrition. This view is reinforced by the practice of *prescribing* these drinks, often on the advice of a dietitian.

Nasogastric and intravenous feeding appear at first glance to be more in the realm of medical therapy. They are invasive and require expertise to accomplish safely and effectively. Are we, however, simply being confused by the sophistication of the intervention? One could take the view that the intended outcome is simply to provide the patient with the food they require in order to continue living. The paraphernalia associated with feeding by these routes is a necessary but morally irrelevant encumbrance.

In the legal case of Anthony Bland, a man in persistent vegetative state who was kept alive by nasogastric feeding, the Official Solicitor argued that ANH was distinct from medical treatment, since it was a basic necessity of life, without which he would die.[13] It was contended that doctors had a continuing duty to provide food and hydration to the patient, and that to discontinue them constituted manslaughter or even murder. In response, the House of Lords took a view similar to that given with regard to the 'three square meals' given to Jodie – that the continuance of life for Anthony Bland was dependent on a comprehensive medical regime, of which nutritional support was an inseparable part. The appropriateness of continued feeding was judged on the basis that it is medical therapy, not basic care. As such it might be withdrawn or withheld like any life-prolonging treatment, where commencing or continuing it was not in the patient's best interests. One must conclude from this that the sophistication of a feeding intervention determines its legal status. Interestingly it does not appear to directly settle its moral worth.

NUTRITION AS MEDICAL TREATMENT

If nutrition is to be afforded the legal status of medical treatment, the process of decision making surrounding its use becomes a therapeutic decision, similar to that invoked when deciding the appropriateness of antibiotic therapy or surgery, for example. In this situation it becomes necessary to consider the objectives of therapy and the wishes of the patient concerned.

Objectives of therapy

Before commencing a therapeutic regime, it is usual to consider the end-points one is trying to achieve, and nutritional support has an impact on at least four outcomes:

1 prolonging life
2 creating health
3 preventing disease
4 relief of symptoms and palliation.

Before considering the moral significance of these objectives, it is important to decide whether or not they can be achieved. This requires consideration of two further factors:
1 could nutrition achieve the objective for any patient?
2 could nutrition achieve the objective for this particular patient?

It may be difficult to provide answers to these questions. Evidence in support of the hypothesis that nutrition achieves an objective in particular circumstances is often lacking or of poor quality. Health workers may have to draw on their own experiences. The absence of high-quality evidence does not necessarily invalidate the subjective conclusions of a team of experienced professionals. It is more important that an effort is made to assess the best available evidence, and that the values of individuals do not contaminate such evidence. The latter situation may occur when an individual seeks to bias, suppress or ignore evidence in order to influence the final decision. The second question involves assessment of the prognosis, a process which is also imprecise and subjective. Consider, for example, the following case.

CASE 4.2

Ged is dysphagic following a stroke. He is assessed by the stroke unit as having a 'reasonable' prognosis for good functional outcome. His doctor is aware of research evidence suggesting a benefit from the early use of PEG feeding following such a stroke. A request is made to the endoscopy service, but the endoscopist refuses on the basis that although the procedure is reasonably safe, the quoted evidence is of low quality. He also remarks that Ged's prognosis is 'appalling', and that he would not want a PEG tube for any relative of his with a stroke.

Comment
In this case the endoscopist is choosing to ignore evidence that the PEG tube might help Ged, in the absence of any clear evidence that it would definitely harm him. He is also introducing imprecise estimates of prognosis. Such views appear to be driven at least in part by the values of the endoscopist, who is opposed to PEG feeding for stroke patients in general. Failure to remain objective while assembling evidence of benefit or harm will confuse discussion of the values attached to various therapy goals. This is arguably a failure of professional duty to the patient.

Having taken care to assemble the best evidence, and to make the best estimate of prognosis, it should be possible to ascertain the likelihood of achieving various objectives. In practice, objectives will be met to a greater or lesser degree, and it is helpful to estimate where the therapy lies on the spectrum between success and failure.

For example, consider Figure 4.1.

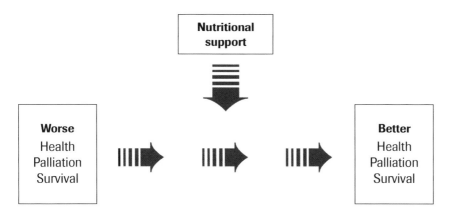

FIGURE 4.1 Estimating where the therapy lies on the spectrum between success and failure

It is now necessary to decide upon the moral worth of each objective, a process which will be influenced both by the circumstances of the patient and by the professional values of those involved in the decision making. If survival is to be valued above all else, then an intervention which has any impact on improving survival will be favoured, even at the expense of poor palliation or compromised patient health. Alternatively, those who value quality of life most highly may be prepared to accept an intervention that provides palliation at the expense of reduced life expectancy.

There are several benefits of this approach. First, it makes the decision-making process explicit and provides an opportunity to separate out the practical elements of a decision (will the therapy work?) from the moral elements (which outcomes are most valued in this case?). Second, it may be employed by all individuals involved in the decision making, first separately and then in committee. Where moral conflict arises, it may be possible to address the problem by making explicit the values attached by individuals to the various therapeutic objectives. Third, although the process requires calculations of the moral worth of various outcomes to be made (i.e. a teleological or outcome-based approach), it also permits a rule-based (i.e. deontological) approach should one choose to value one particular outcome, such as the preservation of life.

The wishes of the patient

If nutritional support has assumed the status of medical treatment, then as with any other treatment it is necessary to seek the consent of that individual before proceeding. Older patients for whom nutritional support is contemplated are often unable to participate fully in the decision making due to their illness, and difficulties arise when the wishes of the patient are not clear. One approach to this situation is outlined in Chapter 3, and the elements of the process are summarised below.

➤ A valid consent to treatment requires that the patient is competent, informed and voluntary.

➤ To have capacity to decide about treatment, a patient should be able to take in and retain information about the proposed treatment, balance the risks and benefits in their own mind and arrive at a choice.

➤ If the patient lacks capacity and cannot take part in the treatment decision, surrogates must decide in a way that is morally justifiable.

Surrogate decision making about nutritional support is not without problems. In a follow-up study of individuals who decided to accept tube feeding for their elderly incompetent relative, two-thirds were satisfied with their decision and four-fifths would do the same again.[14] Even so, almost one-third of relatives in retrospect felt that the patient did not want the tube.

One way to facilitate best interests decisions or create advance statements is to engage older people in discussions about nutritional support in advance of their requiring it. This is of particular importance in those likely to require artificial nutrition, such as patients with dementia or progressive neurodegenerative disease. At present such discussions are not commonplace but appear acceptable to older people, can be presented in an easily comprehensible format (e.g. using vignettes) and do not provoke anxiety.[15] In one large study, only one-third of competent older individuals in nursing homes would elect to have a feeding tube in the event that they suffered brain damage and were unable to eat.[16] An advance decision or properly appointed welfare attorney may provide the information about what a patient now lacking capacity would have wished in these circumstances. If none is available, family members may provide vital information on cultural, religious and personal beliefs that may affect the decision on whether to feed an individual artificially.

NUTRITION AS BASIC CARE

If nutritional support assumes the status of basic care, decision making about its use is often driven by beliefs which surpass those employed in making a therapeutic decision. In particular, it is the values which are attached to continued comfort, well-being and ultimately life which enable the correct course of action to be decided upon.

A framework which adheres to these values is set out in the ancient Jewish ethico-legal system known as *halacha*.[17] In this system, the preservation of life takes precedence over virtually all other considerations. This stems from the belief that God has made man in his own image and in addition has given him the gift of life to be held in trust. Honouring and preserving this life is both a duty and a means of honouring God. Quality-of-life issues are of lesser importance, and only those measures that cause severe pain and suffering are to be avoided, specifically when a patient is moribund or death is imminent. In general, however, nutritional support, by whatever means, should not be refused or withdrawn, since to do so would hasten the patient's death.

Others who take a more moderate approach might view ANH as an 'extraordinary' measure which might be refused in situations where the patient is irreversibly and terminally ill. For example, patients with advanced dementia who have impaired swallowing may be considered terminally ill, given a median survival of only six months. Other moral frameworks have also employed the distinction between 'ordinary' and 'extraordinary' care in deciding about life-sustaining treatment. Care is extraordinary and therefore not obligatory if it involves great cost, pain or burden to the patient or to others, without reasonable chances of success.[18] Here the argument hinges on what one considers to be a success. If it is purely the maintenance of life, then life-sustaining care may be classed as ordinary. If success means more than this, perhaps the restoration of full health, then painful or costly care which does not meet this objective is considered extraordinary.

Opponents of this approach take the view that what is costly, painful or otherwise burdensome today might be cheap and trouble-free in the future. Indeed, the relative ease with which ANH can now be undertaken has arguably led to its becoming 'ordinary' care, whereas a decade ago it might have been considered 'extraordinary'. Others might argue that because the objectives of care determine its moral status, it is not the care which requires evaluation but its end-points. According to this view it is less important to distinguish medical therapy from basic care, and more important to decide upon the value of the possible end-points.

The most extreme *halachic* view might override the values of the patient, perhaps on the grounds that no individual has the right to refuse that which gives life. Others would consider refusal only on the basis that it would prolong suffering and that otherwise every second of life is infinitely precious. In general, however, classifying nutrition as basic care removes some of the barriers to decision making which might otherwise encumber patients and their relatives when attempting to participate in a strictly medical decision. The complexity of medical decision making arguably makes it a less accessible process, whereas decisions based on values may be more equitable.

SHOULD WE FEED THIS OLDER PATIENT?

As there is often no clear evidence of whether ANH is appropriate in a given situation, an ethical framework can support the decision-making process. The framework (*see* Table 4.1) does not provide a comprehensive guide to all the arguments which might be mounted in favour of or against feeding, but may be used to give structure to the complex process of evaluating a particular case. It allows all interested parties to be involved.

TABLE 4.1 An aid to decision making around the provision of artificial nutrition and hydration

For use in patients in whom reversible factors such as missing dentures, intercurrent illness or depression have been excluded
Arrange meeting with family, carers and members of the multidisciplinary team • Is there evidence of an advance decision? • Explore understanding and explain about underlying medical condition and likely prognosis. • Consider and discuss what the patient is likely to have wanted in this situation. • Try to consider cultural, religious and personal beliefs.

Decision made to NOT provide ANH	**Decision made to provide ANH**
• Continue to hand feed where possible. • Provide high-quality mouth care. • Provide high-quality palliative care when appropriate. • Remain in communication with the family, reviewing if necessary.	• Set objective goals with family. • Agree timescale for review – suggest 2–4 weeks.

If unable to make a decision . . . • Ask for a second opinion. • Consider use of independent advocates. • Consider a time-limited trial of ANH.

As with all morally important decisions, the outcome should be reviewed regularly to ensure that both the circumstances and the values on which the decision was based have not altered significantly over time. Where the decision was not to feed, this will involve rehearsing once more the arguments already outlined.

Once the decision has been taken to feed a patient, there are a number of additional factors to be addressed prior to discontinuing feeding.

SHOULD WE STOP FEEDING THIS OLDER PATIENT?

Discussions about stopping feeding will occur when it is apparent that continuing to feed is not the correct course of action. In practice, this may occur for one of three reasons:
1   patient circumstances have changed
2   the values of those involved have changed
3   issues relevant to the decision were not considered.

Patient circumstances have changed

Where objectives of care can be met without nutritional support, perhaps because of improved patient prognosis, stopping feeding will not be problematic. Examples include recovery of swallowing following a stroke, or restoration of consciousness following delirium.

Difficulties will arise when the passage of time creates a clearer understanding of patient prognosis, leading to a change in the objectives of care. This may occur when the patient deteriorates or fails to show any signs of improvement. The following two cases illustrate these problems.

CASE 4.3

Peter was admitted to hospital following a stroke three months ago. Because of swallowing difficulties, a PEG tube was inserted for feeding purposes. Despite comprehensive attempts at rehabilitation, he has made no progress and one week ago suffered a second stroke which has left him unconscious but otherwise clinically stable.

CASE 4.4

Cathy has learning disability and was living in a residential home prior to admission. One month ago she developed septicaemia following a perforation of her colon. Following surgery to remove bowel, IV feeding was commenced to correct malnutrition and facilitate recovery. Despite attempts at rehabilitation, she has remained fully dependent on nursing care.

In the case of Peter, the objectives of feeding included maintenance of life and good functional outcome from his stroke. Recent events indicate that the latter objective is unlikely to be met, and discussion must now centre on the value attached to his continued living, together with any new objectives such as palliation of distressing symptoms. Meanwhile Cathy is unlikely to achieve functional independence, although she shows no signs of further deterioration. Here the objectives of care must alter. Rather than restoring functional independence, feeding is only likely to maintain present stability. Discussion of the appropriateness of continued feeding must therefore involve evaluation of these new or reprioritised objectives. While discussion here may focus on conversion to a less sophisticated means of feeding (such as PEG) it is nevertheless opportune to examine the values which underlie all forms of feeding rather than dwell simply on its delivery mechanism. In practice, it is all too easy to ignore values and settle decisions purely on the clinical grounds.

The values of those involved have changed

Having gained experience of the effects of feeding over a period of time, those involved in the decision to feed may choose to alter the values they originally attached to objectives. For instance, the original decision may have been based on an overwhelming desire to maintain continued life, which has subsequently given way to the more valued objective of preventing distress. This is illustrated by the following case.

CASE 4.5

Joyce was left with speech and swallowing difficulties following evacuation of a subdural haematoma two months ago. After discussion with her daughter and in her best interests, it was decided to insert a PEG tube to facilitate feeding. Despite attempted rehabilitation she has made no progress and remains dependent for all nursing care. She has acquired pressure sores and grimaces in pain when moved. Her daughter now feels that the need to preserve life does not justify Joyce's continued suffering.

When a decision has been reached by carers and relatives together, a sustained change in values of one person should prompt re-evaluation of the decision by all members of the team. This will again ensure that the basis of any new decision is explicit and based on clear objectives of care. For example, the views of Joyce's daughter may alter if she is reassured that her mother's pain can be adequately controlled and that continued feeding may help her pressure sores.

Particular difficulties may arise when the values of the patient become altered by the passage of time – for instance, when a patient no longer wants nutritional support. Here it is helpful to retrace the decision-making process with the patient to clarify the basis of their new decision and to evaluate their competence to do so. In certain circumstances, legal clarification may be required. This is illustrated by the following case.

CASE 4.6

June has suffered from Parkinson's disease for eight years and has become severely malnourished. Three months ago she consented to have an NG tube inserted to facilitate feeding. Despite adequate feeding, she has remained fully dependent and is awaiting admission to a nursing home. She has now decided that she does not wish to live in this condition, and has made a refusal of further feeding via the tube.

Given that unconsented touching may constitute battery or assault, the legal implications of June's refusal for her carers are significant. Evaluating her decision making may clarify whether she has the capacity to refuse feeding, and may elucidate the values on which she bases her refusal. This will help her carers to decide on what basis they must either respect her wishes or override her refusal. If June has capacity, then her wishes must be respected even if malnutrition ultimately results in her death.

KILLING OR LETTING DIE?

No decision about nutritional support will be free from the elements of this debate, which centres on the moral equivalence of the acts which constitute killing and omissions which result in death.[18] Consider the following case.

CASE 4.7

Jeremy suffered a stroke one year ago which left him unable to swallow, and a PEG tube was inserted. He now states that he wishes to die and requests that the tube be removed. This would require an endoscopic procedure, which the endoscopist refuses to undertake on the grounds that his actions would ultimately lead to Jeremy's death. Instead he recommends that the tube be left in place but not used. Jeremy's nurse argues that this has the same effect and that he does not wish to stand by and watch his patient die by his omission.

The endoscopist believes that an action which leads to Jeremy's death has more moral weight than an omission which leads to the same outcome. He could argue that removing the tube causes Jeremy's death, and that he is therefore killing him by agreeing to his request. He could also argue that he is assisting in Jeremy's suicide or even that his actions constitute active voluntary euthanasia. The nurse, on the other hand, does not draw a distinction between an act or

---

omission, on the basis that the outcome is the same. His argument might focus on whether or not it is right for Jeremy to die, not on the means by which this outcome could be achieved.

One could argue that without the PEG tube, Jeremy's death would be inevitable, and the tube is merely a barrier to events for which his carers are not responsible. Tube removal does not constitute killing him; it is simply allowing him to continue his journey towards death. Others might argue that we are obliged to remove the tube out of respect for Jeremy's autonomy. In this case his death may be foreseen, but it is not an intended effect of our actions, simply a side-effect.

Alternatively, one could argue that we have a duty to care for Jeremy, which includes providing effective barriers to his death. If we do not prevent his death, then we might also decide not to prevent the deaths of others. This might place us on a 'slippery slope' towards withholding treatment for all patients who are dying. Furthermore, as carers we have a duty to care, but not to undertake activities which compromise our own moral standards. We are not obliged to do something to Jeremy which might lead directly to his death, even if he demands it.

There is no right or wrong solution to this dilemma, but it is important that those involved in such difficult decisions are individually comfortable with the outcome. There is no substitute to working through the arguments, guided by the frameworks outlined previously. This will not only lead to a morally robust decision, but will also facilitate discussion in those difficult cases where legal clarification is the only way forward.

The law

In English law, the majority of cases dealing specifically with nutrition have centred on the tube feeding of individuals without their consent, or the withdrawal of tube feeding from individuals unable to express their views. Some of the key issues are summarised below.

➤ Food is legally identified by its chemical composition, not by its form of administration.
➤ Liquid food does not therefore constitute medicine.
➤ Artificial feeding does, however, form part of a regime which amounts to medical treatment.
➤ Medical treatment generally may not be administered to a competent adult without their consent.
➤ In the case of incompetent adults, feeding decisions should follow their best interests.

Assessment of best interests usually includes discussion with family members.
➤ There is no obligation to give treatment that is futile or excessively burdensome.
➤ The law regards withholding or withdrawing treatment as an 'omission', not an 'act'.
➤ When contemplating forced feeding or withdrawal, seek legal clarification.

KEY POINTS

- A decision to artificially feed an older person requires consideration of the benefits, feasibility and morality of the proposed procedure.
- The objectives of nutritional support should be evaluated by estimating the likelihood of success.
- The wishes and values of the patient must be considered, either contemporaneously or in the form of advance statements.
- For patients who are unable to express a view, a morally robust feeding decision may emerge after wider consultation.
- Decisions to commence feeding should be reviewed in the light of changing patient circumstances or values.
- Decisions to stop or to impose feeding create complex moral problems which may require legal clarification.

REFERENCES

1 Department of Health. *Improving Nutritional Care: a joint action plan from the Department of Health and Nutrition Summit Stakeholders.* London: Department of Health; 2007.
2 McWhirter JP, Pennington CR. Incidence and recognition of malnutrition in hospital. *BMJ.* 1994; **308**: 945–8.
3 Incalzi RA, Capparella O, Gemma A, *et al.* Inadequate caloric intake: a risk factor for mortality of geriatric patients in the acute care hospital. *Age Ageing.* 1998; **27**: 303–10.
4 Kagansky N, Berner Y, Koren-Morag N, *et al.* Poor nutritional habits are predictors of poor outcome in very old hospitalized patients. *Am J Clin Nutr.* 2005; **82**: 784–91.
5 Anderson CF, Motness K, Meister J, *et al.* The sensitivity and specificity of nutrition-related variables in relationship to duration of hospital stay and rate of complications. *Mayo Clin Proc.* 1984; **59**: 477–83.
6 British Geriatric Society. *Guidelines on Artificial Hydration and Nutrition in Elderly Patients.* Document G1. London: British Geriatric Society; 1977, revised 2003.
7 Gillick MR. Rethinking the role of tube feeding in patients with advanced dementia. *NEJM.* 2000; **342**: 206–10.
8 Haddad RY, Thomas DR. Enteral nutrition and enteral tube feeding: review of the evidence. *Clin Geriatr Med.* 2002; **18**: 867–1.

9 Grant MD, Rudberg MA, Brody JA. Gastrostomy placement and mortality among hospitalized Medicare beneficiaries. *JAMA*. 1998; **279**: 1973–6.

10 Mitchell SL, Kiely DK, Lipsitz LA. The risk factors and impact on survival of feeding tube placement in nursing home residents with severe cognitive impairment. *Arch Intern Med*. 1997; **157**: 327–2.

11 General Medical Council. www.gmc-uk.org

12 British Medical Association. www.bma.org.uk

13 *Airedale NHS Trust v Bland* (1993) 1 All ER 821.

14 McNabney MK, Beers MH, Siebens H. Surrogate decision makers' satisfaction with the placement of feeding tubes in elderly patients. *J Am Geriatr Soc*. 1994; **42**: 161–8.

15 Ouslander JG, Tymchuck AJ, Krynski MD. Decisions about enteral tube feeding among the elderly. *J Am Geriatr Soc*. 1993; **41**: 70–7.

16 O'Brien LA, Siegert EA, Grisso JA, *et al*. Tube feeding preferences among nursing home residents. *J Gen Intern Med*. 1997; **12**: 364–71.

17 Schostack Z. Jewish ethical guidelines for resuscitation and artificial nutrition and hydration of the dying elderly. *J Med Ethics*. 1994; **20**: 93–100.

18 Harris J. *The Value of Life*. London: Routledge; 1985.

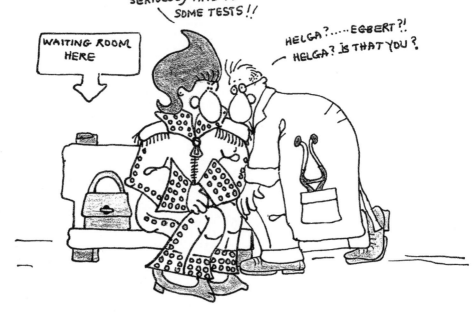

CHAPTER 5

Communication, barriers to it and information sharing

David Oliver and Philippa Gee

WHY GOOD COMMUNICATION MATTERS AND WHAT OLDER PEOPLE WANT

Effective communication between professionals and patients is inherent to a moral duty of beneficent care and in respecting patients' right to autonomy over their own treatment.[1] As the common law on consent to treatment,[2] the Mental Capacity Act 2005[3] the Adults with Mental Incapacity (Scotland) Act 2000[4] all recognise, adequate information is a pre-condition of informed decision making. The Parliamentary Enquiry into the Human Rights of Older People in Healthcare[5] identified inadequate communication as a potential threat to Article 3 (the right to prohibition of cruel or degrading treatment) and Article 14 (right to freedom from discrimination) under the European Convention 2008.[6]

Good communication includes a duty to offer patients: diagnosis and prognosis, including limits of knowledge; treatment options; implications and side-effects of treatment; main alternatives and the opportunity to ask questions. Older patients have identified these elements as key – for example, in studies on older people's views on end-of-life care,[7] which emphasised the central importance of communication in treatment planning, with many older people wanting active involvement in planning their own treatment. Better communication can also aid concordance with medical treatment.[8,9]

Good reciprocal communication involves establishing a relationship in which patients feel empowered to ask questions or raise concerns of their own. They should be able to decide the amount of detail and style of information they want, have control over decision making, including any delegation, involvement of family members, or in some cases the wish to be shielded from bad news. Some older people may be culturally deferential to professionals and inhibited about questioning doctors but professionals should find out what patients want to know and how they want it communicated.

While patients' beliefs, values and culture can affect what they choose to ask and how they handle information, blanket assumptions should not be made about what individuals might want, based solely on their age, background or ethnicity. All patients should be initially encouraged to be involved in decision making. Deliberate concealment of facts that patients want to know, or covert medication of competent people, is an abuse of human rights. While these considerations matter for all patients, older people are at especial risk of communication failure.

HOW COMMUNICATION WITH OLDER PATIENTS CAN FAIL AND POTENTIAL BARRIERS TO GOOD COMMUNICATION

As patients get older they are less likely to receive the right treatment, adequate information or discussion of treatment options and they may be seen as a stereotype based on a set of assumptions based on age alone. If on top of this they have problems with hearing, eyesight or cognition, if they are frail and if they have no strong advocate, they are at risk of being marginalised in decisions about their treatment

When older people or their families discuss 'dignity in care',[10] many issues relate to 'insufficient choice' and 'not being listened to or treated as an individual'.[11] In European focus groups on dignity,[12] poor communication and information giving were seen by older people as key threats to their dignity. Concrete examples of dignity being compromised included being 'patronised', 'excluded from decision making' and 'treated as an object'. So why is this likely to happen?

Older patients are more likely to have physical disability or frailty, cognitive, hearing or visual impairment, so styles of communication and information more suited to younger, fitter patients may not always be appropriate and older patients may not be so able or ready to ask professionals for different or more information. Conversely, professionals may make patronising and ageist assumptions about the amount of information or decision making that older people should be afforded and fail to communicate to a degree that would seem a bare minimum in younger patients.[13] For instance, Adelman, et al.[14] found that doctors provided more information, were more supportive and more willing to share decision making with younger rather than older patients and that those patients were often reluctant to challenge them.

Professionals may also fail to see older people as individuals with individual values and communication needs, viewing them merely as a category – 'elderly people'.[7] This may be compounded by misguided attempts to 'protect' older patients from frank discussion, motivated either by paternalistic intentions to act in their 'best interests' or because the health professional fears being perceived as 'insensitive' or attracting complaints from family members.

Some staff have especial difficulties in dealing with older patients from ethnic minorities – a 'disabling hesitancy'[15] – or in staff from one ethnic background dealing with older people from another. Kai, *et al.*[15] concluded that while better awareness and training might help in providing culturally sensitive communication, the onus is still on staff to treat older patients as individuals.

All these factors may result in diagnosis, treatment or future care arrangements being discussed behind the older person's back, or with their families only, while the older person is effectively denied the right to determine their own future care or to take risks.[16,17] This can be compounded by social attitude, expectations or beliefs of the family. Families are often central to providing care for their elders, but might believe that paternalistic, family decision making is in the older person's best interests and that older people should not have the same right to self-determination or information about their condition as younger people.[18]

The phenomenon of 'elder speak' has been described by Williams, *et al.*[19] and is something we can all recognise. Here, staff employ infantilising language – which could further reinforce dependency and helplessness – as well as insulting the older person's human dignity. As Williams, *et al.*[19] concluded, '. . . the messages of dependence, incompetence and control to older adults by using elder-speak, a speech style similar to baby talk, that fails to communicate appropriate respect'.

They describe elder speak thus: 'typically the rate of speech is slower, louder, more high pitched and using more exaggerated intonation than normal adult speech. Repetition, simple vocabulary and simple grammar are also facets of this way of talking. Diminutives and intimate terms of endearment are used rather than individuals' names'.

All of this reinforces the concerns raised by older people in the various reports on dignity and rights.[11,12,7,4] Repeatedly in these reports, the issues are raised of: inadequate information; inadequate help, time or sensitivity in the delivery of that information; inadequate consideration of the humanity of the older person as an individual; inadequate mechanisms to allow older patients to express their views and preferences or to discuss their worries; and inadequate respect for the decisions they wish to make over their own care.

PRACTICAL SUGGESTIONS TO IMPROVE COMMUNICATION WITH OLDER PATIENTS TO MEET THEIR OWN NEEDS, EXPECTATIONS AND THE EXPERIENCE AND EFFECTIVENESS OF CARE

Much of the advice on improving communication follows from the issues set out below. The list is not exhaustive but key points include:

1 *The need for appropriate, individualised, person-centred, non-ageist communication, including amount and form of information*

Older people will have individual expectations, and others should not make blanket assumptions based on age, gender, illness, disability or ethnicity. Some older people freely express a wish to devolve decision making to trusted family members or professionals or not to be burdened with much information about their treatment, illness or prognosis. In these circumstances it is misguided and maleficent to force full and frank communication. Nonetheless, the older person should retain the right to express his or her own concerns or questions or to receive 'basic' information to a degree which suits their individual needs. If there are cultural considerations, these should be addressed in a culturally sensitive manner. And if barriers to communication are identified (see below), then strategies should be devised in partnership with patients or carers to overcome these for that individual.

Research has repeatedly shown[20,7,21] that older people's preferences are generally far more in favour of full information giving than health professionals or their families anticipate (even in cultures where collectivist and family decision making is the norm). Both professionals and family can be overcautious about causing upset. Education and training can overcome such attitudes and improve skills in the communication with older people in general[22] and with elders from ethnic minorities.[23]

With regard to elder speak, there will be occasions where information needs to be simplified in order to make it accessible to the patient. The onus is on the professionals to make such information simplified but not simplistic.

2 *The use of written information, in some circumstances*

This is not a substitute for adequate verbal communication. But it may help for those whose first language is not English, those with poor short-term memory or poor retention due to anxiety, and those with hearing impairment. The use of such information may increase satisfaction with care and understanding of treatment, reduce complaints, improve self-care and management and make the older patient feel more empowered, so reducing their anxiety or distress.[24]

3 *Interpreters*

While most hospitals and primary care organisations have access to interpretation services, staff sometimes rely on family members or friends.[11] This can cause problems when there are no immediate family or friends and might potentially compromise the privacy and dignity of the older person if sensitive personal information is being shared with others merely because of the ease of an 'on hand' translator. It might be hard for those personally involved to translate impartially if they themselves have views, agendas, vested interests or control over that older person. Booking an external interpreter may sometimes be impractical where instant communication is required, but this option should always be available to older patients. If hospital staff are used as *ad hoc* interpreters, it is preferable that they are clinically trained rather than ancillary staff.

4 *Services for the hard of hearing*

The Royal National Institute for Deaf People[25] estimates that there are 123 000 deafened people over 16 within the UK, with the incidence of deafness increasing with age. We often fail to consider whether an older person in health or social care settings has a hearing loss, whether diagnosed or undiagnosed – with the assumption being made that they don't understand, are confused or are simply being obstructive. Yet The Mental Capacity Act[3] states that capacity should always be assumed unless proven otherwise. Professionals have a duty to facilitate adequate understanding and information giving. This entails an obligation to perform adequate assessment and remediation if possible of any hearing loss. Deaf people who communicate using sign language can also exhibit the characteristics of aphasia following a stroke.[26] Difficulty in communicating is further compounded by the use of elder speak, as shouting can distort the pattern of speech and the use of high-pitched tone exacerbates the situation as the hearing loss pattern associated with ageing is so often one of high-frequency loss.[27]

5 *Patients with dysphasia*

Dysphasia or aphasia may be defined as 'a complex disorder which can affect comprehension, speech, reading and writing to varying degrees' and impacts on approximately one-third of stroke survivors.[28] It often co-exists with other disorders such as hearing loss, visual impairment, dysarthria and dyspraxia. It is often assumed that older people with aphasia cannot understand or communicate sufficiently well to make decisions – thus increasing their vulnerability.[29] The Connect Report[28] stated that: 'People with aphasia are frequently treated as stupid. They can feel excluded, ignored and unable to participate fully in life. And that's on top of the personal struggle of learning to live with a long term disability.'

Older people with a possible diagnosis of aphasia should be formally assessed to determine the degree of disability and be given the chance fully to participate in any decision making even if this requires facilitation.[30,31]

6 *Patients with dementia/cognitive impairment*

Once patients have a diagnosis leading eventually to mental impairment, unjustified assumptions are often made about their ability to process information and only limited attempts are made to communicate. Patient groups[32,33] have expressed concerns that staff can automatically make assumptions and set low expectations about the ability of older patients with dementia to communicate or make care decisions, even though the literature on mental capacity[34,35] and the legal tests[3] make it clear that the mere presence of the diagnosis does not make the older person incapable of decision making or of some involvement in planning their own care.

Unless assessment of an individual's mental capacity demonstrates impaired cognition, people should be offered information in a way they can best comprehend it. Where assessment shows that the patient lacks mental capacity, relatives, carers or others close to the person should be consulted to throw light on what the incapacitated person would have wanted. The recent Bournewood Ruling from the European Court of Human Rights[36] made it clear that even for adults with mental incapacity, full access should be allowed to their social network and as much autonomy over their own care as is feasible.[37]

The final responsibility for making treatment decisions rests with the health professional in charge if they are acting exclusively out of concern for that older person's best interests. When invoking 'best interests', the Department of Health 2007[17] and the guidance accompanying the Mental Capacity Act 2005[3] still prioritise communication, encouraging the following elements:

➤ doing whatever is practical to help the person participate in decision making
➤ identifying factors that the person would take into account if acting for him or herself
➤ reflecting his or her known wishes and any statement made before capacity was lost
➤ identifying the values that would be likely to influence the decision if the patient had capacity
➤ avoiding assumptions about his or her best interests based on age, appearance, condition or behaviour
➤ considering whether he or she is likely to regain capacity and
➤ consulting other people where possible for their views.

7 *Patient advocates and witnesses to discussions*
Health professionals may be suspicious of recorded or witnessed consultations, seeing them as a breach of trust or a potential threat of litigation. Nonetheless, they can be helpful for some older patients to ensure that advice is remembered accurately, though it may alter the nature of the conversation. Professionals may be less willing to speculate about future options or explore areas of uncertainty with patients when the conversation is recorded. Having a relative or patient advocate present helps some patients if they have

hearing or communication problems or if English is not their first language. As long as patients agree, it is good practice to involve people close to them, bearing in mind the duty of confidentiality. This can also help carers meet the individual's care needs. Competent patients should be offered a choice about who is involved in the discussion.

Patient advocacy services are provided by some charitable organisations and public services providers such as local authorities and National Health Service (NHS) hospitals, in order to help individuals understand the choices available to them and to represent their views and concerns. Legally, patient advocates (even independent mental capacity advocates appointed under the Mental Capacity Act[3]) have no formal decision-making powers, but can help the decision-making process by facilitating communication. Advocates should be properly trained and whether or not an advocate is present, health professionals should, where possible, still communicate directly with the patient as patients accompanied by advocates or carers feel excluded if health professionals fail to speak directly to them. There are times when an independent advocate with no emotional investment in the situation is the most appropriate person to support a person making difficult decisions. However, roles must be clearly defined and everyone involved needs to be aware of the scope and limits of advocates' powers.

INFORMATION SHARING

We have discussed above the need for adequate, appropriate and individualised communication with older people. However, in many cases where their needs are complex it is impossible to plan their care without sharing information and discussing details of their case. Sometimes, it will be in an older person's best interests to discuss aspects of their care with family or friends. And where optimum care of an older person requires input from a range of agencies and professionals, a degree of information sharing between professionals and agencies is desirable and inevitable.

Reports have shown[38,36,39,40] that many older people actively wish information to be shared between agencies and resent having to repeat the same information to several professionals. They are quite happy to have information shared, so long as it is between individuals acting for their welfare. For all this, there are caveats and concerns around information sharing.

Areas of law relevant to information sharing in the care of older people

The following are some key relevant areas of law which concern information sharing.

➤ *Data Protection Act 1998.*[41] This requires organisations fairly and lawfully to process information on patients and provides that patients must know what information about them is being processed. The processing must meet legal standards for confidentiality. The Act also requires organisations sharing information to share the *minimum necessary* and to retain this only or as long as is needed.

All *identifiable, patient-related* information is subject to a professional duty of confidentiality. Electronically stored or written information must be protected and stored securely. Any confidential conversations should be conducted out of earshot of others. However, there are exceptions to these rules:
— where the patient gives consent to others being informed
— where the law requires disclosure of information
— where there is an overriding public interest.

➤ *Human Rights Act 1998, Article 8.*[42] This articulates a right to 'respect for private and family life', though this right is not absolute and may be derogated from where necessary in a democratic society in the interests of national security, public safety, economic well-being or the prevention of crime.

➤ *Common law.* This reinforces the view for various judgments that information may be disclosed with patient consent, where there is a public interest or where the law requires it.[2]

➤ *NHS care record guarantee.* This sets out rules governing information held electronically by NHS care records, including patients' access to own records and control over access by others.

➤ *Professional codes of conduct.* These set out duties around confidentiality, privacy and data sharing.[43,44]

➤ *Internal policies of employing organisations.* All patients who are mentally competent have a right to object to the disclosure of information that they provide in confidence.

Patient consent to disclosure may be implicit or explicit. When health professionals make implicit assumptions, they must demonstrate that they were acting in good faith in assuming consent.

INFORMATION SHARING WITH PATIENTS' RELATIVES

This is a common area of misunderstanding and conflict between healthcare staff and patients' relatives. Relatives and carers often object to being excluded from day-to-day discussion of a patient's care. In complaints from the relatives of older patients, concerns are often raised that 'we were given no information/ were not told what was going on' – even where the older patient was lucid and fully able to discuss their own care. This suggests an ageist assumption in society, that older people should somehow have information about their progress proactively shared with families (or even friends, neighbours and informal carers), even without any formal request for this or acknowledgement of the older patients' wishes or permission. Were we to apply such attitudes to young or middle-aged patients, they would seem morally impermissible.

Of course, many older patients *do* want their families to be kept informed, but all patients are entitled to confidentiality and should first be asked about if and how they want information shared with other people. Although patients often assume that their spouse or other close relatives will automatically be included in information sharing, they need to make their own wishes clear. Health professionals cannot assume that patients are necessarily on good terms with their relatives or want them to have confidential information, unless explicit provision has been made for that.

A further communication problem arises when relatives insist that *they alone* be given information without its being shared with the patient – even in relation to patients who are mentally competent and in cases where there might be potentially useful treatment options which the older patient could be offered, if they were informed of them.

The law and information sharing with patients' relatives and friends

Information on mentally competent patients should not be shared with family members without their consent. It is *for the patients to decide* what information is shared and with whom. Where patients lack capacity, it is usual to assume that they would want those close to them to be informed, unless there is clear evidence that they would not want information shared or it becomes evident that to share information would put the patient at risk.

INFORMATION SHARING WITH OTHER PROFESSIONALS

Poor communication between care providers is a frequent cause of serious adverse events in healthcare. A breakdown in the communication of data, such as investigation results, can be due to a lack of clarity or prior agreement about who has ownership of the data and the responsibility for ensuring that other health professionals are kept informed. Help the Aged[7] gathered examples of lack of co-ordination/communication between healthcare staff or between healthcare providers and social care staff – especially when older patients were discharged from hospital or transferred from one type of care to another. Evidence of poor communication between health staff also occurred in hospital settings when the health professionals providing specialised care had been informed about the patient's need for that specialised treatment but had not been given other relevant information, such as the fact that the patient was blind or suffered from dementia. The National Institute for Health and Clinical Excellence has particularly highlighted the need for well-organised dementia care.[45] Research also shows that 'much of the distress experienced by people with dementia and their families can be prevented when primary care works closely with geriatric nurse practitioners and community and voluntary services'.[46] Such working in partnership is the expected norm for various facets of caring for older people and it does require good communication.

The law and information sharing with other professionals

In the absence of evidence to the contrary, patients are generally assumed to have consented that information be shared with other professionals for the purpose of the care they receive, so long as that information is both *necessary* and *relevant*. It is important that patients know what information will be shared and with whom. This has implications for older people with *multi-agency working*, including social services, housing associations, voluntary agencies, etc. Health professionals should discuss with patients from the outset the desirability of such information sharing.

Other relevant specific points of law around data sharing

The law and secondary use of information

If information is being used for research, audit or service planning, it may be disclosed to an appropriate authority if:
➤ it is sufficiently anonymised
➤ it is required by law
➤ it is with explicit consent
➤ health professionals are satisfied that the patient is aware of its use and has not objected (implied consent)
➤ health professionals are satisfied that legal and professional criteria for disclosure 'in public interest' have been met.

The law and data sharing in official complaints

Here it is implicit that a complaint cannot be satisfactorily answered without adequate access to information, though there is guidance from health departments on confidentiality in complaints.

The legal position on information sharing in summary

➤ Patients must be properly informed about the use of information.
➤ Consent should be sought for disclosure of personal information.
➤ Occasionally where consent can't be obtained, information may be disclosed where the law requires it or where there is a public interest.
➤ Health professionals should anonymise information wherever possible.

➤ Health professionals should disclose the minimum needed to achieve the purpose.
➤ When competent patients refuse disclosure, their wishes should be respected.
➤ Health professionals should always be able to justify the reason for their disclosure.

CONCLUSIONS

Good communication between clinicians, patients, their families, carers and other professionals or agencies is crucial in the delivery of high-quality care. This is all the more important when the older patients are frail, disabled, have sensory or cognitive impairment or complex needs. Yet it is often with these very patients that communication and confidentiality can be compromised. High-quality care should provide individually tailored communication which respects human dignity, as well as known attitudes and beliefs, and gives the patient autonomous control over decisions affecting their healthcare. While the role of family and carers is often crucial to safe care of such older patients, it is very important that the wishes and views of older people are not bypassed in favour of family members or carers. It is also true that effective care often does require communication between agencies and professionals. Nonetheless, in sharing such information, it is important that the older person retains some control over the extent and detail of such sharing and that information is shared only to the extent that it will benefit the care of the older person in question. An awareness of these issues and the ethical and legal considerations which surround them is crucial in the day-to-day clinical and social care of older people.

REFERENCES

1 Gillon R. Medical ethics: four core principles plus attention to scope. *BMJ.* 1994; 309: 184–6.
2 Mason JK, McCall Smith RA, Laurie GT. Consent to treatment. In: JK Mason, RA McCall Smith, GT Laurie (eds). *Law and Medical Ethics.* 6th ed. London: Lexis Nexis; 2002. pp. 309–64.
3 *Mental Capacity Act 2005.* London: Office of Public Sector Information. Available at: www.opsi.gov.uk/ACTS/acts2005/ukpga_20050009_en_1 (accessed 14 April 2009).
4 *Adults with Incapacity (Scotland) Act 2000.* London: Office of Public Sector Information. Available at: www.opsi.gov.uk/legislation/scotland/acts2000/asp_20000004_en_1 (accessed 14 April 2009).
5 House of Lords, House of Commons Joint Committee on Human Rights. *The Human Rights of Older People in Healthcare.* London: Office of Public Sector Information; 2007.

6 *Human Rights Act 1998.* London: Office of Public Sector Information. Available at: www.opsi.gov.uk/ACTS/acts1998/ukpga_19980042_en_1 (accessed 14 April 2009).

7 Help the Aged. *Listening to Older People: opening the door for older people to explore end of life issues.* London: Help the Aged; 2006.

8 British Medical Association. *Evidence Based Prescribing.* London: BMJ Publishing; 2007.

9 Engova D, Duggan C, MacCallum P, *et al.* Patients' understanding and perceptions of treatment as determinants of adherence to warfarin treatment. *Int J Pharm Pract.* 2002; **10**(suppl): R69.

10 Aitken M. The dignity and privacy of patients. *J Royal Soc Med.* 2008; **101**(3): 108–9.

11 Healthcare Commission. *Caring for Dignity: a national report on dignity in care for older people while in hospital.* London: Healthcare Commission; 2007.

12 Woolhead G, Calnan M, Dieppe P, *et al.* Dignity in older age: what do older people in the United Kingdom think? *Age Ageing.* 2004; **33**: 165–70.

13 Oliver D. Acopia and social admissions are not diagnoses: why older people deserve better. *J Royal Soc Med.* 2008; **101**(4): 168–74.

14 Adelman R, Greene M, Charon R, *et al.* Content of elderly patient–physician interviews in the medical primary care encounter. *Communication Research.* 1992; **19**(3): 370–80.

15 Kai J, Beavan J, Faull C, *et al.* Professional uncertainty and disempowerment responding to ethnic diversity in healthcare: a qualitative study. *PloS Medicine.* 2007; **4**(11): 323.

16 Counsel and Care. *The Right to Take Risks.* London: Counsel and Care; 1993.

17 Department of Health. *Independence, Choice and Risk: a guide to best practice in supported decision-making.* London: Department of Health; 2007.

18 Edwards H, Chapman H. Communicating in family aged care dyads; the influence of role expectation. *Quality in Ageing.* 2004; **5**(2): 3–9.

19 Williams K, Kemper S, Hummett ML. Enhancing communication with older adults: overcoming elderspeak. *J Geront Nurs.* 2004; **30**(10): 17–25.

20 Ajaj A, Singh MP, Abdulla AJJ. Should elderly patients be told they have cancer? Questionnaire survey of older people. *BMJ.* 2001; **323**: 1160.

21 Scriven MW. Patients' attitudes towards 'do not attempt resuscitation' status. *J Med Ethics.* 2008; **34**: 624–6.

22 Baltes MM, Neumann EM, Zank S. Maintenance and rehabilitation of independence in old age: an intervention programme for staff. *Psychol Aging.* 1994; **9**(2): 179–88.

23 Cancer Research UK. *Professionals Responding to Cancer and Ethnic Diversity (PROCEED).* London: Cancer Research UK; 2006. Also available at: http://info.cancerresearchuk.org/proceed (accessed 14 April 2009).

24 Payne SA. Balancing information needs: dilemmas in producing patient information leaflets. *Health Informatics J.* 2002; **8**: 174–9.

25 Royal National Institute for Deaf People. *Impact Report.* London: RNID; 2008. Available at: www.rnid.org.uk

26 Royal College of Speech and Language Therapists. *Communicating Quality 3.* London: RCLST; 2006. Available at: www.rcslt.org/resources/ (accessed 14 April 2009).

27 Kulkarni K, Hartley DE. Recent advances in hearing restoration. *J Royal Soc Med.* 2008; **101**(3): 116–24.

28 Connect. *No Longer Invisible: Connect's impact report.* London: Connect; 2006. Available
    at: www.ukconnect.org
29 Hilari K. Predictors of health-related quality of life in people with chronic aphasia.
    Aphasiology. 2000; **17**(14): 365–81.
30 Royal College of Physicians of London, Intercollegiate Working Party on Stroke.
    National Clinical Guidelines for Stroke. London: Royal College of Physicians; 2008.
31 Rose M. The effectiveness of aphasia-friendly principles for printed health educa-
    tion materials for people with aphasia following stroke. *Aphasiology.* 2003; **17**(10):
    947–63.
32 The Scottish Dementia Working Group is an independent group run by people with
    dementia. Available at: www.alzscot.org/pages/sdwg/sdwgcontact.htm (accessed 14
    April 2009).
33 Department of Health. *The National Dementia Strategy.* London: Department of
    Health; 2008. Available at: www.dh.gov.uk/en/SocialCare/Deliveringadultsocialcare/
    Olderpeople/NationalDementiaStrategy/index.htm (accessed 14 April 2009).
34 Alderson P, Goodey C. Theories of consent. *BMJ.* 1998; **317**: 1313–15.
35 Grisso T, Appelbaum P. Comparisons of standards for assessing patients' capacities
    to make a treatment decision. *Am J Psychiatry.* 1995; **152**: 1033–7.
36 Department of Health. *Briefing Sheet. Mental Health Bill. Bournewood safeguards.*
    London: Department of Health; 2006.
37 Harwood RH, Stewart R, Bartlett B. Safeguarding the rights of patients who lack capac-
    ity in general hospitals: do the Bournewood proposals for England and Wales help
    or hinder? *Age Ageing.* 2007; **36**: 120–1.
38 Department of Health. *The National Service Framework for Older People.* London:
    Department of Health; 2001. Available at: www.dh.gov.uk/en/Publicationsandstat
    istics/Publications/PublicationsPolicyAndGuidance/DH_4003066 (accessed 14 April
    2009).
39 Healthcare Commission, Audit Commission, Commission for Social Care and
    Inspection. *Living Well in Late Life.* London: Office of Public Sector Information;
    2006.
40 *With Respect to Old Age: the Royal Commission into Long Term Care for Older People.*
    London: HMSO; 1999.
41 *Data Protection Act 1998.* London: Office of Public Sector Information.
42 *Human Rights Act 1998.* London: Office of Public Sector Information. Available at:
    www.opsi.gov.uk/ACTS/acts1998/ukpga_19980042_en_1 (accessed 14 April 2009).
43 General Medical Council. *The Duties of a Doctor Registered with the General Medical
    Council.* London: General Medical Council; 2006.
44 Nursing and Midwifery Council. *Professional Conduct: standards for conduct, perform-
    ance and ethics.* London: Nursing and Midwifery Council; 2006. Available at: www.
    nmc-uk.org/aFramedisplay.aspx?documentID=201 (accessed 14 April 2009).
45 National Institute for Health and Clinical Excellence. *Dementia: supporting people
    with dementia and their carers in health and social care.* NICE Clinical Guideline 42.
    London: NIHCE; 2006. Available at: www.nice.org.uk/guidance/cg42 (accessed 14
    April 2009).
46 Downs M, Bowers B. Caring for people with dementia. *BMJ.* 2008; **336**: 225–6.

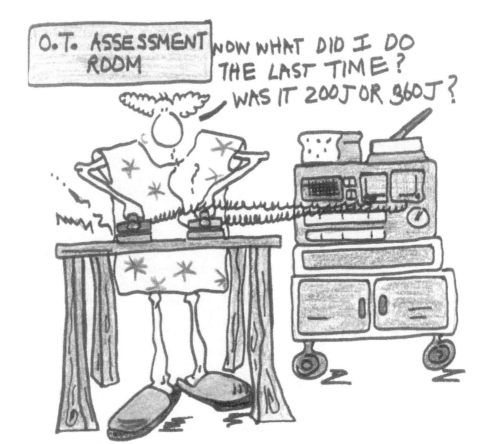

CHAPTER 6

Cardiopulmonary resuscitation

Kevin Stewart and Gurcharan S Rai

INTRODUCTION

Cardiopulmonary resuscitation (CPR) is routinely attempted when hospital inpatients suffer cardiac arrest, unless a specific decision is made in advance to withhold it. However, such 'do not attempt resuscitation' (DNAR) decisions can be controversial. In the UK, there has been considerable press and public concern about DNAR decisions following several high-profile cases, and there have been demands for more openness and transparency in the decision-making process. In 2007, the British Medical Association (BMA), the Royal College of Nursing and the Resuscitation Council (UK) updated their guidelines on DNAR decision making to take into consideration the Mental Capacity Act 2005 (England and Wales), the Adult with Incapacity (Scotland) Act 2000 and provisions of the Human Rights Act 1998. The articles of the Human Rights Act 1998 which pertain to decision making about resuscitation include:

➤ Article 2 – the right to protection for life
➤ Article 3 – the right to freedom from inhuman or degrading treatment
➤ Article 8 – the right to respect for privacy and family life
➤ Article 10 – the right to hold opinions and receive information
➤ Article 14 – the right to be free from discriminatory practices (e.g. ageism).

The guidelines recognise that:
1 the goal of medicine is not just to prolong life at all costs
2 it is lawful to withhold CPR on the basis that to do so would be in the patient's best interests, where consideration has been given to relevant medical factors and the quality of life of patients who lack capacity
3 a competent patient has the right to accept or refuse resuscitation after he or she has been fully informed of its benefits and risks

4 it is not necessary to initiate discussion with patients if there is no reason to believe that they are likely to suffer a cardiopulmonary arrest

5 doctors should always be prepared to discuss DNAR decisions with competent patients and they should usually consult other staff

6 under the Human Rights Act 1998, relatives and carers have the right to information with the consent of the competent patient. Their role is to help the doctor in decision making and to reflect what the incompetent patient would choose in the current circumstances, if competent. They do not have the right to demand or reject resuscitation or a DNAR order

7 in case of adults who lack capacity, the clinician should use the guidance included in the Mental Capacity Act 2005 in assessing best interests

8 The overall responsibility for decisions about CPR and DNAR rests with the consultant or general practitioner in charge of the patient's care.

MAKING A DNAR DECISION

When should a DNAR decision be made and on which patients?

Predicting which hospital inpatients might require DNAR decisions is difficult. Most of those patients who survive CPR attempts have a cardiac arrest within the first couple of days of hospital admission, but at this time many patients may be too ill to be involved in decision making. Studies suggest that around 40% of acute medical inpatients may lack capacity to make such decisions.

It is considered appropriate to make a DNAR decision in the following five circumstances:

1 where the clinical outcome, including the likelihood of successfully starting the patient's heart and breathing, is poor

2 where CPR is not in accord with the recorded, sustained wishes of a competent patient

3 where successful CPR is likely to be followed by a length and quality of life which would be unacceptable to the patient

4 where the patient already has a poor quality of life and does not wish to have his or her life prolonged

5 where the patient has made an advance decision refusing CPR under a clearly defined situation.

Who should make the decision?

'Senior experienced doctors' should take responsibility for decision making. In hospital practice in the UK, this is likely to mean those at consultant or specialist registrar level, or those with similar experience. In some circumstances it may be necessary for more junior staff to make decisions, such as when they are the most senior doctor attending a deteriorating patient who has a very clear advance refusal of life-sustaining treatment. In such circumstances good practice guidance suggest that more senior doctors are informed of the decision as soon as practicably possible.

If there is doubt or disagreement about decisions, full active treatment should be given until the situation is resolved.

DISCUSSION WITH THE PATIENT AND FAMILIES

Competent patients

The guidelines recommend that all DNAR orders on competent patients should be discussed with them, unless they indicate that they do not want this. It may be acceptable to avoid such discussion if it is considered that this is likely to be harmful to the patient (i.e. cause anxiety and distress). Doctors who avoid discussing decisions with competent patients in these circumstances must be able to explain their decisions on the basis that the potential for harm justifies excluding the patient from the process.

Discussion of CPR should focus on:

➤ the risks and benefits of CPR for the individual, with a realistic estimate of the chances of starting the heart and breathing for a sustained period and the likelihood of long-term survival and associated morbidity
➤ the patient's wishes, feelings, beliefs and values
➤ the patient's human rights, including the right to life and the right to be free from degrading treatment
➤ the likelihood of the patient's experiencing severe unmanageable pain, suffering or other adverse effects.

In cases where discussion with the patient is likely to be harmful, or if the patient is too ill to express a view, the doctor must decide using the principle of best interests outlined in the Mental Capacity Act 2005 (England and Wales).

If a patient becomes incompetent after they have made a decision, then their original decision stands provided that the circumstances which have arisen are as envisaged by them when they made the decision. Clearly if a long period of time has passed since the initial decision, then there is a risk that circumstances may have changed significantly. It is recommended that DNAR and other such decisions are reviewed regularly to avoid this problem.

Incompetent patients

If the patient is not competent and has not left clear instruction (in the form of an advance decision or nominated a proxy decision maker using the lasting power of attorney), or does not have a Court-appointed deputy or guardian, then the doctor has an obligation to act 'in the best interest' of the patient (*see* Table 6.1). In practice, this means discussing the decision (where practicable) with other professionals involved in the patient's care, the patient's family, others close to them and any formal or informal carers.

Such discussions should not focus on asking family and friends to act as proxy decision makers (the doctor still has an obligation to make the decision) but should seek to determine the patient's best interest. To do this, the doctor might ask about the patient's previously held views and beliefs or any statements which they may have made in the past. Questions such as 'What do you think your father would have wanted for himself if he knew he was going to be in these circumstances?' may be useful in the discussion.

TABLE 6.1 Factors to be taken into account when making a 'best interests' assessment

- Identifying things that an individual would take into account if acting for himself or herself

- The patient's past and present expressed wishes

- The patient's beliefs and values

- Views of family, friends, carers and GP regarding what the patient would have wanted for themselves

- Views of an independent mental capacity advocate if the patient has no family or friends.

DIFFERENCES OF OPINION BETWEEN PATIENTS AND THEIR FAMILIES

Conflict between the view of patients and that of their families can arise under several circumstances.

1 If a competent patient refuses to give permission to doctors to discuss his or her medical condition and treatment options – under these circumstances, the patient's views prevail.

2 If the decision made by the competent patient is different to that suggested by the relatives – under these circumstances, the physician should facilitate a discussion between them with the aim of reaching a common understanding of the rights of competent patients to exercise their autonomy.

3 Families sometimes question patients' competence (or doctors' assessment of this), especially perhaps when they disagree with DNAR decisions which apparently competent patients have made. In these circumstances doctors should carefully record their assessment of competence using a standardised approach and the questions suggested by the guidance to the Mental Capacity Act 2005. Second clinical opinions can help to clarify the situation in disputes around competence.

WHEN THE SUCCESS OF CPR IS CONSIDERED TO BE POOR

Although the term 'medical futility' is not included in the guidelines, it is recognised that a clinical team need not attempt CPR if the team believes that it
will not re-start the heart and maintain breathing or if a patient is in his or her
final stages of a terminal illness. If, however, a person wishes to delay death,
even for a short period, this wish should be respected provided this has been
made after full, accurate information has been provided to about the length of
survival that realistically can be expected.

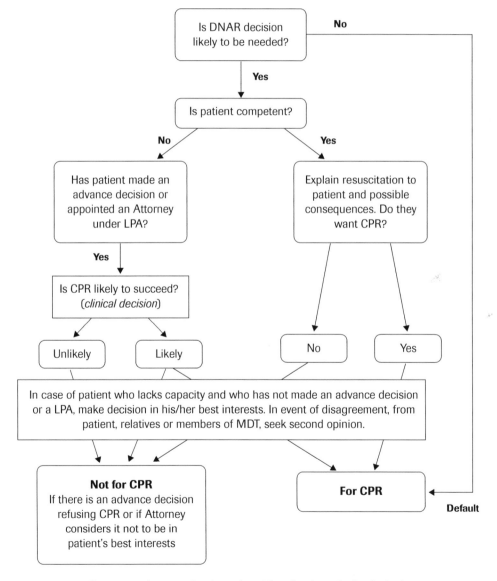

FIGURE 6.1 Suggested resuscitation algorithm for hospital admission

CASE 6.1

Mrs A, aged 84 years, was admitted to hospital with intracerebral bleeding following a fall. She had a past history of manic-depressive illness and required supervision from her husband for basic activities of daily living. At the time of admission she had a Glasgow Coma Score of 9/15, and had spontaneous movement in the left arm and left leg but no movements in the right leg and right arm and bilateral plantar extensor responses. The duty medical registrar who assessed Mrs A made a DNAR decision on the grounds that CPR was unlikely to be successful and would not be in her best interests. However, when he discussed this with Mrs A's husband and daughter, they demanded that she should be resuscitated. Despite a prolonged discussion, no consensus could be reached.

A second clinical opinion was sought from an experienced colleague. He agreed that CPR was unlikely to be successful and undertook further discussion with the family. He discovered that they feared that a DNAR order would mean Mrs A's being denied access to tube feeding, antibiotics and other life prolonging treatment. When it was explained to them that this was not the case, they accepted the need for a DNAR order.

Comments

1 Patients' families and some professionals, may believe that a DNAR decision automatically precludes other life-prolonging treatments. DNAR decisions refer to CPR only.
2 Second clinical opinions can help to clarify situations and resolve differences of opinion with families.
3 It is often difficult to be sure that CPR will not succeed unless patients are clearly in the last few hours of life. If there is a degree of uncertainty about this, and there is no other basis for making a DNAR decision, then they should remain for CPR until the situation becomes clearer.

CASE 6.2

An 84-year-old woman with longstanding rheumatoid arthritis, who required a considerable amount of aid and support from the community services, was admitted with a one-week history of nausea and vomiting. She was somewhat dehydrated but otherwise clinically stable. She seemed mildly confused and her Abbreviated Mental Test Score (AMTS) was 7/10. No family were present when she was admitted. The middle-grade doctor who admitted her concluded that it would be difficult to resuscitate her successfully should she have a cardiorespiratory arrest, and recorded DNAR in her notes. He did not discuss this with the patient.

Comments

Several issues arise from this case.

- It appears that an assumption was made that the patient was incompetent. While many acute medical inpatients may be incompetent, a competence assessment should be documented if decisions about life-prolonging treatment are being made.
- If decisions are being made about patients who are assumed to be incompetent, then efforts should be made to elicit the opinions of family and friends around their best interests.
- Doctors in training or those who are relatively inexperienced should be cautious about making decisions about CPR, or other life-prolonging treatments, without reference to senior colleagues.
- Unless the clinical situation is grave, or rapidly deteriorating, then it is often best to avoid making DNAR decisions early after admission when the information available in likely to be incomplete.

FURTHER READING

Appelbaum PS. Assessment of patients' competence to consent to treatment. *NEJM.* 2007; **357**: 1834–80.

British Medical Association. *The Impact of the Human Rights Act 1998 on Medical Decision Making.* London: British Medical Association; 2000.

British Medical Association. *Decisions Relating to Cardiopulmonary Resuscitation: a joint statement from the British Medical Association, the Resuscitation Council (UK) and the Royal College of Nursing.* London: British Medical Association; 2007.

Department of Health. *Mental Capacity Act 2005.* London: Department of Health. Available at: www.justice.gov.uk

General Medical Council. *Withholding and Withdrawing Life-Sustaining Treatments: good practice in decision making.* London: General Medical Council; 2002.

O'Keefe S, Redhan C, Keane P, *et al.* Age and other determinants of survival after in-hospital cardiopulmonary resuscitation. *Q J Med.* 1991; **81**: 1005–10.

Raymont V, Bingley W, Buchanan A, *et al.* Prevalance of mental incapacity in medical inpatients and associated risk factors: cross sectional study. *Lancet.* 2004; **364**: 1421–7.

Stewart K, Spice CL, Rai GS. Where now with do not attempt resuscitation decisions? *Age Ageing.* 2003; **32**: 143–8.

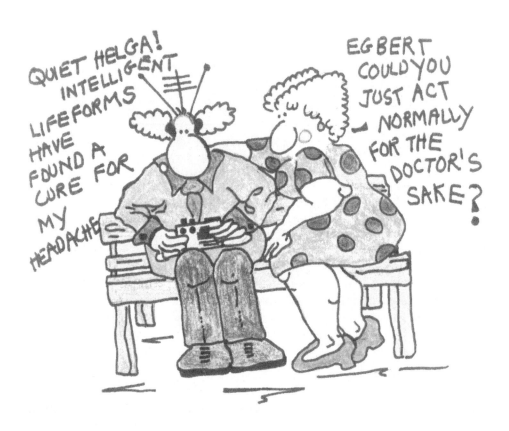

CHAPTER 7

Mental capacity and best interests

Steven Luttrell

The right of a mentally competent adult to refuse medical or any other intervention is enshrined in the Mental Capacity Act 2005 and reinforced by the Human Rights Act 1998, which incorporates the European Convention on Human Rights into domestic law. The Mental Capacity Act codifies and adds to a large number of common law decisions on capacity and has made this area of law considerably more accessible to both doctors and the public. Guidance on the application of the Act is set out in the Mental Capacity Act Code of Practice, details of which are highlighted in this chapter.

A person may refuse treatment for reasons which are 'rational, irrational or for no reason', and a doctor may be liable for assault or battery or for breach of Article 8[*] of the Convention on Human Rights if they touch a person contrary to his or her wishes. However, if the person is mentally incapable, whether temporarily or permanently, the doctor has a duty to act in his or her patient's best interests.

A decision on mental capacity is ultimately a question of law for a court to decide. However, most decisions about mental capacity for the purpose of making a call about medical treatment options never reach lawyers and are undertaken by the treating doctor. As a result of the prevalence of dementia, cerebro-vascular disease, delirium and depression in older people, mental incapacity is a significant issue for doctors.

PRINCIPLES

The Mental Capacity Act, based on over a decade of work undertaken by the Law Commission, is underpinned by a set of five key principles. These are set out in Section 1 of the Act:

---

[*] Article 8 of the Human Rights Act is the right to private and family life, and also incorporates the right to protect the physical integrity of a person.

(i) a presumption of capacity – every adult has the right to make his or her own decisions and must be assumed to have capacity to do so unless it is proved otherwise

(ii) individuals being supported to make their own decision – a person must be given all practicable help before anyone treats them as not being able to make their own decisions

(iii) unwise decisions – just because an individual makes what might be seen as an unwise decision, they should not be treated as lacking capacity to make that decision

(iv) best interests – an activity done or decision made under the Act for or on behalf of a person who lacks capacity must be done in their best interests, and

(v) least restrictive option – anything done for or on behalf of a person who lacks capacity should be the least restrictive of their basic human rights and freedoms.

ASSESSING MENTAL CAPACITY

The 2005 Act sets out a clear test for assessing capacity (*see* Section 2(1)). The assessment is both decision and time specific and is based on the common law judgments set out in the *Re C* (1994),[1] a case in which the High Court was asked to decide whether a schizophrenic patient from Broadmoor Hospital was mentally competent to refuse amputation of a gangrenous leg, and the Court of Appeal case *Re MB* (1997),[2] concerning a young pregnant woman.

In assessing capacity, two questions should be asked:

1 Does the person have an impairment of the mind or brain, or is there some sort of disturbance affecting the way their mind or brain works? (It does not matter whether the impairment or disturbance is temporary or permanent.)

2 If so, does that impairment or disturbance mean that the person is unable to make the decision in question at the time it needs to be made?

The impairment or disturbance does not have to be permanent and a person can lack capacity to make a decision at the time it needs to be made, even if the loss of capacity is partial or temporary and the capacity changes over time. The assessment is specific to the decision being undertaken and a person with borderline capacity may be able to make simple decisions concerning treatment of a straightforward nature, but unable to make a decision on a more complex issue.

The question 'is the person mentally incapable?' should be answered on the balance of probabilities (i.e. is it more probable than not that the patient lacks the required mental capacity?). Everyone is presumed to be mentally capable until proved otherwise. However, once it is proved that a person is mentally incapable there is a presumption that this continues until the contrary is established.

In answering the question of whether the person is unable to make the decision, you should seek to understand whether the person:

> has a general understanding of the decision that they need to make and why they need to make it
> has a general understanding of the likely consequences of making or not making this decision
> is able to understand, retain and weigh up the information relevant to the decision
> can communicate their decision (by talking, using sign language or any other means).

Relevant information must include what the likely consequences of a decision would be and also the likely consequences of making no decision at all. In some cases, it may be enough to give a broad explanation in simple language; in others, more detailed advice might be required. The more grave the consequences, the more important that the person understands the information relevant to the decision. Information should be presented in a way that is appropriate to meet the individual's needs and circumstances and it is important to use the most effective form of communication for that person.

Section 3(3) of the Act sets out that people who can retain information for a short while must not automatically be assumed to lack capacity and that it depends on what is required for the particular decision in question. Items such as notebooks, photos, posters or recordings can help people to retain information.

In cases where mental capacity is severely impaired, the assessment may be straightforward. However, where impairment is mild or moderate, the assessment is often difficult. In such cases, you should make a comprehensive examination of mental function, having regard to abnormalities in behaviour, language, mood, thought, perception, insight, cognition, memory, intelligence or orientation which may result in an inability to make decisions. You should also be aware of visual, auditory and language impairment which might affect your assessment or the ability of the person to make a decision. Evidence from other members of the multidisciplinary team, especially nursing and therapy colleagues, and from the patient's relatives or friends, may be invaluable in assisting you to come to a decision on capacity.

You should take the following steps to minimise those reversible factors which reduce capacity:

1 treatable medical conditions which affect mental capacity (e.g. acute confusion and depression) should be addressed, and where appropriate the assessment should be delayed until capacity is maximal

2 sensory impairments should be corrected if possible
3 communication aids and support from a speech and language therapist should be considered
4 care should be taken to choose the best location and time for the assessment
5 a decision should be reached as to whether the presence of a friend, relative or interpreter would be helpful.

If faced with conflicts or uncertainty, you should consider whether to seek an independent opinion. The need to seek an independent opinion in difficult cases was set out in guidance in *St George's Healthcare NHS Trust v S* (1998), where it was stated by the Court of Appeal that:

> The authority should identify as soon as possible whether there is concern about a patient's competence to consent to or refuse treatment. If the capacity of the patient is seriously in doubt it should be assessed as a matter of priority. In many such cases, the patient's general practitioner or other responsible doctor may be sufficiently qualified to make the necessary assessment, but in complex cases involving difficult issues about the future health and well-being or even the life of the patient, the issue of capacity should be examined by an independent psychiatrist, ideally one approved under Section 12(2) of the Mental Health Act. If following this assessment there remains serious doubt about the person's competence and the seriousness or complexity of the issues in the particular case may require involvement of the court, the psychiatrist should further consider whether the patient is incapable by reason of mental disorder of maintaining her property or affairs. If so, the patient may be unable to instruct a solicitor and will require a guardian *ad litem* in any court proceedings. The authority should seek legal advice as quickly as possible.

MAKING DECISIONS FOR A MENTALLY INCAPABLE ADULT

Section 1(5) of the Mental Capacity Act sets out the best interest principles. Any act done for or any decision made on behalf of a person who lacks capacity must be done or made in that person's best interest, bearing in mind the requirements of the Act.

Prior to the introduction of the Mental Capacity Act, the law relating to best interests had been developed through a number of common law cases, some of which provoked a substantial amount of controversy. The common law position was most clearly set out in *Re S* (sterilisation: patient's best interests) (2000) 2 FLR 389,[3] where it was proposed that a two-stage test should be applied. The first stage was the application of the 'Bolam test'. This is a legal test applied to negligence law which states that the treatment will be lawful if it accords with practice accepted as proper by a responsible body of medical opinion. It was recognised that this approach may provide the patient with a number of different treatment options. For mentally capable patients, the doctor would proceed to explain the range of alternatives, concentrating on those features of advantage and disadvantage most relevant to the patient's needs and circumstances. This step is not possible for a mentally incapable patient, and in these circumstances the second step is to make a choice on behalf of the person. LJ Thorpe explained this second step by stating:

> In deciding what is best for the disabled patient the judge must have regard to the patient's welfare as the paramount consideration. That embraces issues far wider than the medical. Indeed, it would be undesirable and probably impossible to set bounds on what is relevant to a welfare determination. In my opinion, Bolam has no contribution to make to this second and determinative stage of the judicial decision.

The Code of Practice gives further detailed guidance on the process for making best interest decisions and the factors which should be taken into consideration, and both the Act and the Code add substantially to the previous common law decisions.

In coming to a view on the person's best interests, you should:
➤ do whatever is possible to permit and encourage the person to take part or to improve their ability to take part in making the decision
➤ try to identify all the things that the person who lacks capacity would have taken into account if they were making the decision or acting for themselves
➤ try to find out the views of the person who lacks capacity, including:
(a) the person's past and present wishes and feelings (these may have been expressed verbally, in writing or through behaviours or habits), (b) any beliefs and values, e.g. religious, cultural, moral or political, that would be likely to influence the decision in question, (c) any other factors the person themselves would be likely to consider if they were making the decision or acting for themselves.

You should not make assumptions about the person's best interests simply on the basis of his or her age, appearance, condition or behaviour. You should consider whether the person is likely to regain capacity and whether the decision can wait. You should not be motivated in any way by a desire to bring about the person's death and you should not make assumptions about the person's quality of life.

If it is practicable and appropriate to do so, you should consult other people for their views about the person's best interests and to see if they have any information about the person's wishes and feelings, beliefs and values. In particular you should consult: (a) anyone previously named by the person as someone to be consulted on either the decision in question or on similar issues, (b) anyone engaged in caring for the person, close relatives, friends or others who take an interest in the person's welfare, (c) any attorney appointed under a lasting power of attorney or enduring power of attorney made by the person, and (d) any deputy appointed by the Court of Protection to make decisions for the person. For decisions about major medical treatments or where the person should live, and where there is no one who fits into any of the above categories, an independent mental capacity advocate (IMCA) must be consulted. In undertaking such consultation, you should remember that the person who lacks capacity to make the decision or act for themselves still has a right to keep their affairs private – so it would not be proper to share every piece of information with everyone.

You should also see if there are other options that may be less restrictive of the person's rights.

All of these factors should be weighed in order to come to a decision on what is in the person's best interests.

DEPRIVATION OF LIBERTY

Specific guidance on the deprivation of liberty has been produced in the form of a draft addendum to the Mental Capacity Act Code of Practice. This guidance adds to but does not replace other safeguards in the Act. The guidelines have been drafted in the light of the European Court of Human Rights judgment in the case of *HL v the United Kingdom* (the Bournewood Judgment). This case involved an autistic man with learning disability who lacked capacity to consent to admission to hospital. The European Court held that he was deprived of his liberty and that this was a breach of Article 5(1) of the European Convention on Human Rights. As a result of this judgment, the Mental Capacity Act has been amended to provide additional safeguards. The guidance sets out details of what constitutes 'deprivation of liberty' and any 'managing authority' must seek authorisation from a 'supervisory body' before undertaking to deprive someone who lacks capacity to consent of their liberty within the meaning of Article 5.

The European Court indicated that whether a person is deprived of their liberty depends on the particular circumstances of the case and stated:

> to determine whether there has been a deprivation of liberty, the starting point must be the specific situation of the individual concerned and account must be taken of a whole range of factors arising in a particular case such as the type, duration, effects and manner of implementation of the measure in question.

The distinction between a deprivation of, and restriction upon, liberty is merely one of degree or intensity and not one of nature or substance.

The guidance sets out that the following factors may be considered by the courts to be relevant when considering whether or not deprivation of liberty is occurring:

- the person is not allowed to leave the facility
- the person has no or very limited choice about their life within the care home or hospital
- the person is prevented from maintaining contact with the world outside the care home or hospital.

The guidance sets out ways to reduce the risk of deprivation of liberty. However, it recognises that there may be occasions when depriving a person who lacks capacity of their liberty is necessary to protect them from harm and would be in their best interests. In such circumstances the procedure for seeking authorisation should be used. The Code of Practice sets out when it would be more appropriate to use the Mental Health Act rather than the Mental Capacity Act.

MEDICAL RESEARCH

Details relating to research and incapacity are set out in Chapter 11 of the Code of Practice. The Act applies to research that is intrusive, involves people who have an impairment of, or disturbance in the functioning of, their mind or brain which makes them unable to decide whether or not to agree to take part in the research and is not a clinical trial covered under the Medicines for Human Use (Clinical Trials) Regulations 2004. Research covered by the Act cannot include people who lack capacity to consent unless it has the approval of an 'appropriate body'. In addition it must follow the other requirements of the Act to consider the views of carers and other relevant people, treat the person's interests as more important that those of science and society, and respect any objections a person who lacks capacity makes during research.

In England, the 'appropriate body' must be a research ethics committee recognised by the Secretary of State. Such a body can only approve research if: (a) it is linked to an impairing condition that affects the person who lacks capacity or the treatment of that condition, (b) there are reasonable grounds for believing that the research would be less effective if only people with capacity are involved and (c) the research project has made arrangements to consult carers and to follow the requirements of the Act. In addition, there are two further requirements: either (a) the research must have some chance of benefiting the person who lacks capacity and this benefit must be in proportion to the burden caused by taking part or (b) the aim of the research must be to provide knowledge about the cause of or treatment or care of people with the same impairing condition or a similar one.

KEY POINTS

- The right of a mentally capable adult to refuse medical or any other intervention is enshrined in UK law.
- The law relating to mental incapacity in England and Wales is set out in the Mental Capacity Act 2005 and guidance on its application in the Mental Capacity Act Code of Practice.
- In assessing capacity, two questions should be asked: does the person have an impairment of the mind or brain, or is there some sort of disturbance affecting the way their mind or brain works? If so, does that impairment or disturbance mean that the person is unable to make the decision in question at the time it needs to be made?
- In answering the question of whether the person is unable to make the decision, you should seek to understand whether:
  — the person has a general understanding of the decision that they need to make and why they need to make it
  — the person has a general understanding of the likely consequences of making or not making this decision
  — the person is able to understand, retain and weigh up the information relevant to the decision
  — the person can communicate their decision (by talking, using sign language or any other means).
- If a person is mentally incapable, the decision must be made in that person's best interests.
- In reaching a best interests decision, you should have regard to the previous wishes and feelings of the person and those factors that the person would consider if able to do so. You should also consider the views of others whom it is appropriate and practical to consult.
- In undertaking research involving anyone with mental incapacity, you should have regard to the requirements of the Mental Capacity Act.
- Decision relating to deprivation of liberty should be undertaken in accordance with the Act and the addendum to the Code of Practice.

REFERENCES

1 *Re C* (adult: refusal of treatment) (1994) 1 WLR 290.
2 *Re MB* (1997) 2 FLR 426.
3 *Re S* (sterilisation: patient's best interests) (2000) 2 FLR 389.

FURTHER READING

Mental Capacity Act 2005. Department of Health. Available at: www.justice.gov.uk

Mental Capacity Act 2005. Code of Practice. London: HMSO on behalf of Department of Constitutional Affairs; 2007. Available at: www.justice.gov.uk/guidance/mca-code-of-practice.htm (accessed 15 April 2009).

Mental Capacity Act 2005 Deprivation of Liberty Safeguards. Consultation Paper CP23/07. London: Department of Health; 2007.

Re MB (1997) 2 FLR 426.

St George's Healthcare NHS Trust v S (1998) 3 All ER 673.

The Law Commission. *Mental Incapacity*. London: HMSO; 1995.

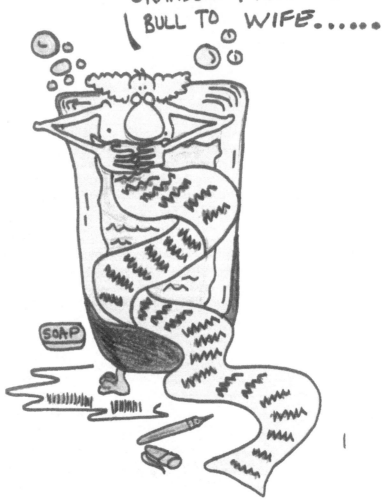

CHAPTER 8

Advance decisions/advance decisions to refuse treatment

Gurcharan S Rai

INTRODUCTION

An advance decision (AD)/an advance decision to refuse treatment (ADRT), otherwise known as an advance directive or a living will,[1] is a statement of treatment preferences that indicates a person's wishes should the capacity for decision making be lost in the future. That is, it sets out clear instruction on refusal of treatment or medical intervention/procedures. Based on the principle of autonomy, it aims to project this forward into possible future mental incapacity.

An advance consent or authorisation similarly defines a person's wishes for advance request for treatment at the time he or she loses capacity for decision making. Unlike an AD, these instructions are not a directive that the doctor has to comply with if it conflicts with his clinical judgement.

BACKGROUND

Advance directives were introduced in the USA following the case of Karen Quinlan. Karen was 21 years of age when in 1975 she developed a permanent vegetative state after taking tranquillisers and alcohol. She was maintained on a respirator with nasogastric feeding. When the Quinlan family realised that there was no prospect of Karen's recovery, they requested that her life support be discontinued. There was no legal precedent for such a decision at that time, and medical opinion was firmly against the proposal. A long legal battle ensued during which the courts involved attempted to determine what Karen's wishes would be in the circumstances then affecting her. In the event, the New Jersey Supreme Court gave permission for Karen to be removed from the respirator.

Ironically, as feeding was continued, it was not until 10 years later that Karen died.

Arising from this and subsequent cases, the view developed that it would be much easier to make decisions in similarly difficult circumstances if the prior wishes of the patient were known. Subsequently, advance directives have been given statutory recognition in all the states in the USA and in Canadian provinces.

A similar debate took place in the UK in the case of Tony Bland, a young man who developed a permanent vegetative state after sustaining injury in the Hillsborough football stadium disaster. Both his doctors and his parents reached the view that after around two years without any improvement in his condition, artificial feeding should be discontinued. The case eventually reached the House of Lords as the highest court of appeal. The Law Lords sanctioned the withdrawal of feeding, and Tony Bland died around four years after being injured.

In giving judgment, a recommendation was made to the effect that Parliament should consider the issues involved. This led to the creation of the House of Lords Select Committee on Medical Ethics, which published its report in 1994.[1] In this report the term 'advance directive' is described as a 'document executed while a patient is competent, concerning his or her preferences about medical treatment in the event of becoming incompetent'. The report commended the development of ADs, but stopped short of recommending statutory legislation to support them, indicating that doctors are increasingly recognising their ethical obligations towards them, and that in any event case law is moving in the same direction.

The report makes important points concerning the implementation of an advance directive:

➤ it may express refusal of any treatment or procedure which would require the consent of the patient if competent
➤ it should not request any unlawful intervention or omission
➤ it cannot require treatment to be given which the healthcare team judge as being not clinically appropriate
➤ such directives could not be given greater legal force without depriving patients of the doctor's professional expertise and the benefit of any new treatments that may have become available since the directive was signed.

This last comment (*see* House of Lords report, paragraph 264) summarises one of the most telling objections to the value of ADs. Instead of legislation, the report recommended that a code of practice be developed by the colleges and faculties of all the healthcare professions to guide their members. This was taken up by the British Medical Association and resulted in the publication of *Advance Statements about Medical Treatment*.[2] The steering group was widely representative of medicine, nursing and the law. In the introduction, the code of practice stated unequivocally that the subject of ADs is quite separate from euthanasia, assisted suicide or allocation of healthcare resources. Such a distinction is clearly not shared universally – witness the support given to ADs by the Voluntary Euthanasia Society.[3] Academics, too, see the subjects as being closely related.[4]

In 1998 the General Medical Council included advice to doctors on 'advance statements' in its document on consent.[5] This is an important step, as it means that awareness of ADs and their observance is mandatory.

The Law Commission, in its report on mental incapacity,[6] recommended specific statutory recognition of advance directives and after long consultation advance directive/refusal was included in the Mental Capacity Act 2005, which came into force in 2007.

ADVANCE DECISION (AD)/ADVANCE DECISION TO REFUSE TREATMENT (ADRT) AND THE LAW

Prior to the coming into force of the Mental Capacity Act 2005, in October 2007, advance decisions to refuse treatment/advance directives were legally valid under common law – the courts recognised that adults have the right to say in advance that they want to refuse treatment if they lose capacity in the future – even if this results in their death. Article 5 of the Act 2005 sets out conditions that must be met for advance refusal/advance directive to be legally valid. These are:

➤ an individual making or drawing up advance refusal must be an adult aged 18 or over
➤ the person must be competent or deemed to be have capacity at the time the AD/ADRT is formulated
➤ the AD/ADRT must specify the treatment that the person wishes to refuse, in medical and lay terms
➤ the person can specify the circumstances in which the refusal will apply
➤ the person making the AD/ADRT has not acted inconsistently with the terms of the refusal
➤ the AD/ADRT must be valid and applicable. It is not valid if it is subsequently withdrawn by the person or by a lasting power of attorney (LPA) appointed by the person. It is not applicable if a person has capacity to make decision at the time of treatment or the treatment has not been specified or if unanticipated circumstances arise which are likely to have influenced the decision
➤ the AD/ADRT dealing with life-sustaining treatment must be written, signed and witnessed and include a statement that the decision applies even if the person's life is at risk
➤ refusal of non-life-sustaining treatment can be verbal.

The Mental Capacity Act 2005 only applies to England and Wales. In Scotland, the area of advance decision making is covered by the Code of Practice issued under the Adults with Incapacity 2000 (Scotland) Act, which advises that an advance decision/directive made by a competent adult should be seen as a strong indication of his or her former wishes. In Northern Ireland, common law applies as there is no statute.

Advance decisions (refusals) made before the Mental Capacity Act 2005

The Act includes transitional and consequential provisions in relation to decisions made before the Act came into force. These transitional provisions accept such decisions, even though they do not comply with the specific recommendation relating to life-sustaining treatment (i.e. they do not include a statement that decision is to apply even if life is at risk with no signature from the person and a witness). The other conditions are:

> the advance decision is in writing
> the person has not withdrawn the decision at a time when they had capacity
> the person does not have the capacity to give or refuse consent to the treatment in question
> the treatment in question and the circumstances are clearly specified in the advance decision
> the clinical staff has a reasonable belief that the AD/ADRT was made before 1 October 2007 and that the person has lacked capacity since that date
> if the doctor believes that the person had the capacity to amend their decision since October 2007, then the above transitional provisions will not apply.

Verbal advance decision to refuse treatment

An individual can make a verbal advance decision to refuse treatment and professionals must follow these if they consider they exist and are valid and applicable, except if treatment is life sustaining – here refusal must be in writing, signed and witnessed.

Advance refusal of life-prolonging treatment

Under the Mental Capacity Act 2005, advance refusal of life-sustaining treatment must be written, signed and witnessed and include a statement that the decision applies even if the person's life is at risk.

Advance refusal of basic care

Basic or essential care – which includes provision of food and water by mouth, warmth, shelter and basic nursing care to keep the person comfortable or to reduce distress such as use of analgesics – cannot be included in an advance statement by an individual. An individual, however, has the right to refuse these measures when offered while they are competent. As and when a patient becomes incompetent, they will still be offered basic care by healthcare professionals for it would be unethical to deny measures to relieve suffering. Having said this, an incompetent person may still refuse to accept fluids or food by not opening their mouth. If refusal is accepted by healthcare professionals as genuine, then physicians must respect this decision.

Advance decisions regarding mental treatment

There is no difference between physical or mental disorder unless a person is detained under the Mental Health Act 1983 and the treatment is being given without consent under Part 4 of the Act.

Protection for professionals from liability

Physicians who do not follow AD/ADRT could face criminal prosecution or be liable to be sued in the Civil Court. The Mental Capacity Act 2005 also provides protection to the healthcare professionals if they withhold or stop treatment because they reasonably believe that a valid and applicable AD/ADRT exists.

CONCLUSION

The ethical basis for AD/ADRT is derived from recognition of individual autonomy. Prior to the Mental Capacity Act 2005, ADs were legally valid under common law. Article 5 of the Mental Capacity Act 2005 sets out conditions that must be met for an AD/ADRT to be legally valid.

KEY POINTS

- An advance decision (AD)/an advance decision to refuse treatment (ADRT), sometimes known as a living will, is a statement of treatment preferences as an indication of a patient's wishes should his or her capacity for decision making be lost in the future.
- AD/ADRT had the authority of common law precedent until the Mental Capacity Act 2005 which came into force in October 2007.
- For AD/ADRT to be valid, an individual must be an adult over 18 years of age, competent at the time, must specify the treatment to be refused and the circumstances in which refusal is to apply.
- AD/ADRT dealing with life-sustaining treatment must be written, signed

and witnessed and include a statement that the decision applies even if the person's life is at risk.

- AD/ADRT prepared before the Mental Capacity Act 2005 came into force in 2007 is valid even if it is not signed or witnessed or contains a statement that the decision applies even if the person's life is at risk, provided the patient has remained incompetent since October 2007.

CASES

CASE 8.I

Mrs A, who is 82 years of age, is admitted with a stroke (total middle cerebral artery infarction) and is not expected to recover. During the hospitalisation, she develops pneumonia for which she is given intravenous antibiotics. Her son, who visits her daily, produces a living will, written on a pre-prepared form. This was prepared six months earlier, after her sister had suffered a stroke. It is signed by Mrs A and witnessed by her general practitioner. In the statement she asserts that she would not wish to be kept alive if she suffered a severe stroke which would leave her dependent upon others for daily care. It is also stated that 'this decision applies even if my life is at risk'.

Comment

This is a valid and applicable advance statement made by an individual who, on probability, was competent at the time she prepared it. Therefore physicians should respect it.

CASE 8.2

A 75-year-old man, Mr B, who has suffered from Parkinson's disease for 15 years and is now experiencing 'on–off' periods and difficulty with speech and swallowing despite changes to therapy recommended by the physician, is admitted with a community-acquired pneumonia and delirium. His wife, who looks after him, informs the physician that her husband is a very religious man and believes that life is sacred and must be preserved at all costs, even if quality seems poor. She requests that all measures including Intensive Therapy Unit (ITU) must be considered.

Comment

No one can demand treatment for himself or herself on behalf of an individual. However, views of a patient made through his or her family members or carers

---

must be respected and used in assessing or planning treatment in his or her best interests, when he or she is no longer competent to make a decision by himself or herself. While an AD/ADRT can be verbal, a vague statement made by the patient does not form the basis of a valid AD/ADRT.

REFERENCES

1 House of Lords. *Report of the Select Committee on Medical Ethics*. London: HMSO; 1994.
2 British Medical Association. *Advance Statements about Medical Treatment*. London: British Medical Association; 1995.
3 Davies J. *Choice in Dying*. London: Ward Lock; 1997.
4 McLean S, Britton A. *The Case for Physician-assisted Suicide*. London: Harper Collins; 1997.
5 General Medical Council. *Seeking Patient Consent: the ethical considerations*. London: General Medical Council; 1998.
6 Law Commission. *Mental Incapacity*. Law Commission Report No. 231. London: HMSO; 1995.

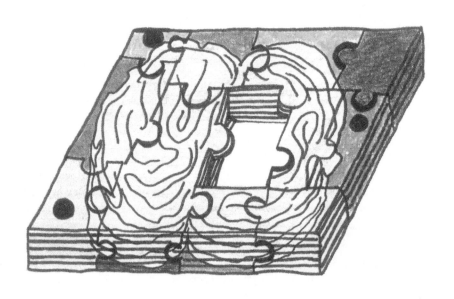

CHAPTER 9

Ethical issues in stroke management

Jonathan Birns and Gurcharan S Rai

BACKGROUND

Stroke is a common condition affecting approximately 150 000 people every year in the United Kingdom, equating to 400–500 people per year in an area served by the average district general hospital. Very few stroke survivors make a complete recovery; 12–18% are left with speech problems, 25% are unable to walk, 50% have residual weakness and 24–53% remain dependent on carers for day-to-day activity.[1] Some 25–30% of patients will die within one month of the stroke and approximately 15% will be residing in institutional care one year after the stroke.

The management of stroke patients involves frequent decisions that require careful ethical consideration. In the early stages, decisions must be made against a background of uncertainty regarding the likely outcome. Later, key decisions are necessary in patients who have been left with severe disability. In addition, many stroke patients are unable to communicate their wishes with regard to treatment and placement decisions.

DIAGNOSIS

An accurate diagnosis is essential when formulating decisions about the management of a patient with an apparent stroke. A number of conditions can mimic the clinical syndrome of a stroke, including an intracranial neoplasm, subdural haematoma, intracranial abscess and hypoglycaemia. In addition, the distinction between cerebral infarction and cerebral haemorrhage cannot be accurately made on clinical grounds alone. The key investigation in establishing the diagnosis is brain imaging, via either a computed tomography (CT) scan or a magnetic resonance imaging (MRI) scan. All patients suspected of having a stroke should have brain imaging performed within 24 hours, in accordance with Royal College of Physicians' guidelines.[2] Although these guidelines are clear, there is often an ethical issue with regard to scanning patients who may have a clinically poor prognosis or multiple disorders where the clinician believes that scanning will not change management or outcome. This may be true in some cases but there are several instances where investigations do not support initial clinical impressions and reveal an element of reversibility. Refusal to perform such a scan on the grounds of age or disability is unethical and all patients should have basic investigations, except in cases where death is imminent and to undertake investigations is likely to cause distress.

PROGNOSIS

Accurate early information regarding prognosis after stroke is crucial to enable rational decisions to be made about a patient's treatment. In a minority of cases it is clear that the patient has a very poor prognosis. For example, a patient with an extensive intracerebral bleed and impending coning or a patient with advanced dementia and a history of several previous strokes has a very poor prognosis. Early decisions to withhold possible life-prolonging measures can be made with confidence in such patients. However, the outlook for most stroke patients is much less clear. While continued assessment provides the best guide for management decisions, a number of approaches can help to provide prognostic information.

Adverse prognostic factors

A number of factors that imply a poor prognosis have been identified in research studies. These include the following:
- unconsciousness on admission
- multiple/severe co-morbidity
- very advanced age
- cognitive impairment
- pre-existing dependence.

Of these, a low level of consciousness on admission is the most secure indication of a poor prognosis.

STROKE SUBTYPES

Intracerebral haemorrhage confers a worse prognosis than ischaemic stroke, with in-hospital and one-year mortality rates being 45–53% for intracerebral haemorrhage and 16–27% for ischaemic stroke respectively.[3] The prognosis for ischaemic stroke is also affected by the stroke subtype. The two most commonly used ischaemic stroke classification systems are the Oxfordshire Community Stroke Project (OCSP)[4] and Trial of ORG 10172 in Acute Stroke Treatment (TOAST) classifications.[5]

The OCSP classification uses clinical localisation of the infarct topography and subdivides strokes into four groups as follows:

1 lacunar infarct – pure motor, pure sensory, sensorimotor or ataxic hemiparesis
2 total anterior circulation infarct (TACI) – higher cortical dysfunction (dysphasia or visuospatial neglect), homonymous visual field defect and hemiplegia and/or sensory deficit involving at least two areas of face, arm and leg
3 partial anterior circulation infarct (PACI) – two of the three components of TACI with higher dysfunction alone or motor/sensory deficit more restricted than those classified as lacunar events
4 posterior circulation infarct (POCI) – ipsilateral cranial nerve palsy with contralateral motor and/or sensory deficit, bilateral motor and/or sensory deficit, disorder of conjugate eye movement, cerebellar dysfunction or isolated homonymous visual field defect.

The TOAST classification denotes five diagnostic subgroups of ischaemic stroke: large-artery atherosclerosis, cardioembolism, small-vessel occlusion (i.e. lacunar stroke), stroke of other determined aetiology, and stroke of undetermined aetiology.

The prognosis for these subtypes is very different. More than 50% of patients with TACI are dead one year after their stroke, and the majority of those who survive a TACI will remain dependent on care to a greater or lesser degree. In contrast, death following a lacunar event is uncommon (less than 10% of cases at one year), and the majority of these patients will regain full independence. Compared with other subtypes, patients with stroke due to large-artery atherosclerosis are three times as likely to have early recurrence within one month[6] and patients with stroke due to cardioembolism or undetermined aetiology have a worse prognosis in terms of disability and mortality.[7]

SCORING SCALES

A number of scoring systems have been developed in order to predict outcome. The most widely used acute stroke scoring system is the National Institute of Health Stroke Scale (NIHSS) that may confer an accurate probability of recovery if used in the first week (*see* Figure 9.1).[8] A score higher than 16 implies a poor prognosis, while one below 6 implies a good prognosis.

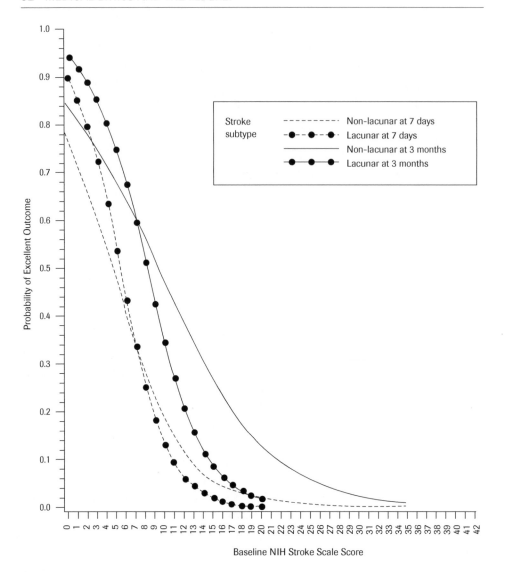

FIGURE 9.1 Probability of an excellent outcome from stroke by NIHSS score[8]

Therefore a number of factors may be taken into account when attempting to provide a patient and their family with accurate information about the likelihood of recovery. An accurate estimate of a patient's chances of improvement also provides a framework to aid decision making. However, it must be remembered that the presentation in an individual patient is key, and that patients who at face value would appear to have a poor prognosis may do surprisingly well.

CASE 9.1

A previously well 69-year-old man was admitted with a dense left hemiplegia. He was semi-conscious with a Glasgow Coma Score (GCS) of 9. A CT scan showed a large basal ganglia bleed with mass effect. Despite the bleed and the low GCS, it was felt that he might do well once the haematoma had resolved. Aggressive supportive treatment including nasogastric feeding and antibiotics was used. The patient's GCS rose to 15 three weeks after admission, and after rehabilitation he was discharged home, requiring only a small amount of help with personal care.

DRUG TREATMENT

Thrombolysis with recombinant tissue plasminogen activator is an accepted form of treatment for acute ischaemic stroke within three hours of stroke onset in selected patients.[9] However, national clinical guidelines advise that thrombolysis should only be administered by personnel trained in its use in a centre equipped to investigate and monitor patients appropriately.[2] Non-administration of thrombolysis to a suitable patient may be regarded by some clinicians as being unethical and national clinical strategies are being developed to ensure that all stroke patients have access to specialist hyper-acute stroke care.[10]

NUTRITION AND HYDRATION

Approximately 45% of stroke patients will have some degree of dysphagia and associated aspiration immediately after their stroke. This will resolve in over 90% of cases during the next three months. Many of these patients will be able to take a soft diet, but some will have a severe degree of dysphagia that precludes oral feeding, and will require an alternative route to be found.

The provision of nutrition and hydration has been regarded as different to the provision of medical treatments. The law regards nutrition and hydration as a basic human right. However, the issue is clouded because both of the means used to provide nutrition and hydration in dysphagic stroke patients (nasogastric tubes and intravenous cannulae) fall under the heading of medical interventions. Thus it can be argued that such treatments (as with any medical treatment) can be provided or withheld at the discretion of the treating medical team, provided decisions are based after full assessment of the individual's case. In practice, virtually no clinician would withhold hydration from a dysphagic stroke patient. However, decisions concerning nutrition are perceived as being more complex because the means used to provide nutrition (nasogastric tubes) is deemed more uncomfortable (and thus less acceptable) than the means used to provide hydration. To complicate matters further, there is a dearth of evidence to guide decisions concerning nutrition, particularly the timing of initiation of enteral feeding. While the FOOD trial demonstrated that early tube feeding may reduce the risk of dying after stroke, the results suggested that improved survival may be at the expense of increasing the chances of poor outcome.[11]

It is generally accepted that withholding nutrition from a stroke patient in the early stages is unethical unless the prognosis is clearly hopeless. Usual practice is to commence nasogastric feeding within 24 hours of admission. Very often patients pull out nasogastric tubes with their good hand, increasing the probability of complications associated with repeated tube insertion. There are also ethical issues surrounding the use of restraint to prevent such patients from dislodging nasogastric tubes (*see* Chapter 13 on restraints). Gastrostomy tubes provide a more secure route for feeding as well as a more reliable supply of nutrition. However, at present there is no evidence to support the immediate use of gastrostomy tubes and their insertion requires a surgical procedure and exposes the patient to potential complications.

Withdrawal of feeding

Withdrawal of nutrition at a later date in a patient who has not improved and who remains very disabled may be an appropriate action. If one regards nutrition via tube feeding as a medical intervention, then according to the medical model, if the indication for such an intervention no longer exists, that intervention can be withdrawn. However, before making a decision on withdrawal of nutrition it is recommended that doctors:

➤ consult the patient if they have the capacity to participate in the discussion, unless death is imminent and discussion with them about benefits, burdens and risks will not be appropriate

➤ consult all members of the healthcare team and those close to the patient

➤ seek a second expert opinion from a senior clinician who has experience of the patient's condition but is not involved in the patient's case

➤ seek legal advice on whether the Court should be involved for a ruling if significant conflicts arise between members of the healthcare team or between the healthcare team and relatives/carers about whether artificial nutrition should be provided.

Withdrawal of feeding is an emotive subject but discussions of this nature may be made much easier if there is appropriate counselling of the relatives before feeding is commenced. It may remain very difficult to withdraw nutrition in a conscious patient because of fears about the symptomatic effects of lack of nutrition and, in practice, nutrition is often continued as a palliative intervention, long after there is any hope of a meaningful recovery.

CHEST INFECTION AND ANTIBIOTICS

The high incidence of dysphagia coupled with other factors – such as reduced mobility, under-nutrition and exposure to hospital pathogens – means that chest infection (and more specifically, pneumonia) is a common problem in patients with acute stroke. In a severely disabled stroke patient, clinicians are often faced with the difficult decision of whether to treat such an infection, or whether it is kinder to withhold medication and allow nature to take its course. The latter decision is difficult to support in the early stages of stroke treatment in view of the problems discussed earlier about initial post-stroke prognostic judgements. One may also note that the administration of intravenous antibiotics is acceptable and generally not distressing to the patient and their relatives, even allowing for the potential side-effects of such agents. Thus, it is common practice (and ethically sound) to treat all such infections in the early stages of stroke management. The situation may be very different if the same patient with the same severe degree of disability develops pneumonia three months later. By this stage, the lack of potential for further recovery is clear and a decision to withhold treatment is ethically and morally supportable.

RESUSCITATION ORDERS

Much controversy exists over the rationale behind the allocation of 'do not attempt resuscitation' (DNAR) orders. The tendency in stroke patients (more than for most other conditions in acute medicine) is for a high proportion of patients to be allocated a DNAR order. This is often done without consultation with the patient or their relatives.

Medically, there are sound reasons why DNAR orders may be appropriate in stroke patients, even in the acute setting. Stroke patients who undergo cardiopulmonary resuscitation (CPR) have been shown to have a reduced chance of survival[12] and concern has been raised about the detrimental effects of the resuscitation process on cerebral perfusion in a patient who is already suffering a degree of brain injury. It is feared that a stroke patient who survives a resuscitation effort will be left with a more severe degree of brain injury and thus greater disability. Furthermore, concern exists over the ability of a stroke patient to survive and be successfully weaned from mechanical ventilation subsequent to initially successful CPR. However, studies of CPR outcome in hospital have often excluded large numbers of stroke patients (because of the frequency with which they are allocated DNAR orders) and thus may not provide a true picture of the potential for survival among such patients. It must also be remembered that stroke patients often have coexistent ischaemic heart disease, which has the potential to cause transient, treatable arrhythmia (e.g. ventricular fibrillation). Further, many stroke patients, particularly those with lacunar infarcts, have a very good prognosis, and issuing such a patient with a DNAR order solely because they have had a stroke is unlikely to be defensible.

Recently updated guidelines[13] issued by the British Medical Association, the Resuscitation Council (UK) and the Royal College of Nursing recommend that:

➤ if a doctor believes that CPR will not re-start the heart and maintain breathing, it should not be offered or attempted

➤ CPR need not be offered when a patient is in the final stages of an incurable illness and death

➤ it is lawful to withhold CPR on the basis that it would not be in the best interests of the patient. Neither the patient, nor his or her family/carers can demand CPR that is clinically inappropriate

➤ if CPR may be successful in re-starting the patient's heart and maintaining breathing for a sustained period, the benefits must be weighed against potential burdens/harms to the patient. However, this decision should consider the patient's wishes/beliefs if he or she has capacity. If such a patient chooses/wants to delay death, even for a very short period, this wish should be taken seriously under the Human Rights Act 1998

➤ in those who lack capacity, decision making must be based in the patient's best interests in line with the Mental Capacity Act 2005.

Finally, it must be understood that a decision not to resuscitate is not the same as a decision not to treat and that issues concerning the administration of antibiotics etc. are quite separate.

CASE 9.2

A 58-year-old man suffered a large intracerebral bleed with a resulting dense hemiplegia, hemianopia and dysphasia. Three months after his stroke, he was transferred to another hospital for further management. No clear decision regarding resuscitation status had been made at the first hospital. A series of difficult interviews were held with the patient's family. The medical staff made clear their view that a DNAR order should be issued. The family was initially opposed to this as they felt that such a decision would be tantamount to killing their relative. However, after many discussions they agreed with the medical viewpoint and the DNAR order was issued.

PLACEMENT

A common problem in the later stages of stroke management concerns issues about the patient's destination on discharge from hospital. Two basic rules are unavoidable. The patient should be discharged to where they wish to go if at all possible, and although this may not always be possible, no patient should be forcibly discharged to somewhere they do not wish to go. The patient's right to self-determination as enshrined in law requires these conditions to be met. Problems arise in those patients who refuse to accept the danger of returning to an unsuitable environment. The law is quite clear about this situation – a mentally competent adult has the right to do what he or she wishes, and the clinician must accede to them.

In cases where concerns exist about the patient's decision-making ability, the patient's mental capacity should be assessed formally in line with the Mental Capacity Act 2005.[14] The Act states that a person is unable to make a decision for himself or herself if he or she is unable:

➤ to understand the information relevant to the decision
➤ to retain that information
➤ to use or weigh that information as part of the process of making the decision, or
➤ to communicate his or her decision (whether by talking, using sign language or any other means).

It should be remembered that a person must be assumed to have capacity unless it is established that he or she lacks capacity and that a person is not to be treated as unable to make a decision unless all practicable steps to help him or her to do so have been taken without success. This is particularly important in stroke patients with dysphasia whose communicative ability is limited. Skilled patient assessment by healthcare professionals, including speech and language therapists, may establish that the patient can communicate their wishes in some way. In such cases, decisions about placement should be delayed until appropriate specialist assessments have been undertaken. It should also be borne in mind that an act done, or decision made, under the Mental Capacity Act for or on behalf of a person who lacks capacity must be done, or made, in his or her best interests.[14]

If a patient lacks capacity for decisions pertaining to discharge, the clinical team must first enquire if, under a lasting power of attorney, the patient has appointed another person to make decisions about the patient's personal welfare, property and affairs.[14] If no such attorney has been appointed, the healthcare team should act in the patient's best interests taking into account the patient's past and present expressed wishes, beliefs and values and the views of their family, friends and carers. The plans made by the healthcare team should be discussed with the patient's family and/or friends to seek their agreement. If the family and/or friends are not in agreement with the care plan or if there is no individual (such as a family member, friend, carer or neighbour) who can act as an advocate, the healthcare team should seek formal advocacy from an independent mental capacity advocate to ensure that the proposed management and discharge planning is in the best interests of the patient.

CASE 9.3

A 78-year-old gentleman, who had previously lived alone, suffered a left middle cerebral artery territory stroke resulting in right-sided neurologic deficits and dysphasia and a dependency on nursing staff for personal care. The members of the healthcare team responsible for his rehabilitation and disability management were in agreement that it would not be safe for this gentleman to return home and that it would be in his best interests to be discharged to a care home. He was assessed as lacking capacity for making decisions about discharge from hospital and had no relatives or friends who could act as an advocate for him. An independent mental capacity advocate was involved to facilitate discharge decisions and they were in agreement with the plan for his transfer to a care home.

DRIVING AFTER STROKE

Legally, patients who have suffered a stroke or transient ischaemic attack should not drive for a month after the event. The patient should be advised to inform the Driver and Vehicle Licensing Authority (DVLA) and their insurance company. After a month, patients may resume driving if this is deemed safe by their clinician. In cases of doubt, an assessment at a Driver Assessment Unit may provide confirmation of a patient's degree of fitness to drive.

Some manifestations of stroke (e.g. homonymous hemianopia) disqualify the patient from driving. The clinician is negligent if they do not inform the patient of this fact, and may be held legally liable should an accident ensue. If a patient who is unfit to drive is known to be continuing to drive and will not inform the DVLA, the clinician can break confidentiality and inform the DVLA himself or herself. In these circumstances, the clinician's responsibility to society outweighs their responsibility to maintain confidentiality.

KEY POINTS

- Only in a very small minority of stroke patients is it possible to state that their prognosis is virtually hopeless within the first few days.
- All patients other than those with no chance of recovery should receive nutrition and hydration, and should have brain imaging performed.
- Withdrawal of treatment may be justified in a patient in whom a poor prognosis has become clearer with the passage of time.
- Other potentially life-saving treatments (e.g. antibiotics) should not be withheld while the prognosis is uncertain.
- It is acceptable to issue a DNAR order while continuing all other treatments.

- It is unacceptable to issue a DNAR order to a patient solely because they have had a stroke.
- The clinician is ethically and legally justified in deciding treatments that are in the patient's best interests for those who cannot express their wishes provided he or she has followed the guidance included in the Mental Capacity Act 2005.
- Communication with patients and relatives at all stages is the best way to ensure acceptability of decisions.

REFERENCES

1 Sacco RL. Risk factors, outcomes, and stroke subtypes for ischemic stroke. *Neurology.* 1997; 49(5 Suppl 4): S39–44.
2 Royal College of Physicians. *National Clinical Guidelines for Stroke.* London: RCP; 2004.
3 Christensen MC, Munro V. Ischemic stroke and intracerebral hemorrhage: the latest evidence on mortality, readmissions and hospital costs from Scotland. *Neuroepidemiology.* 2008; 30: 239–46.
4 Bamford J, Sandercock P, Dennis M, *et al.* Classification and natural history of clinically identifiable subtypes of cerebral infarction. *Lancet.* 1991; 337: 1521–6.
5 Adams HP Jr, Bendixen BH, Kappelle LJ, *et al.* Classification of subtype of acute ischemic stroke. Definitions for use in a multicenter clinical trial. TOAST. Trial of Org 10172 in Acute Stroke Treatment. *Stroke.* 1993; 24: 35–41.
6 Lovett JK, Coull AJ, Rothwell PM. Early risk of recurrence by subtype of ischemic stroke in population-based incidence studies. *Neurology.* 2004; 62: 569–73.
7 Pinto A, Tuttolomondo A, Di Raimondo D, *et al.* Risk factors profile and clinical outcome of ischemic stroke patients admitted in a Department of Internal Medicine and classified by TOAST classification. *Int Angiol.* 2006; 25: 261–7.
8 Adams HP Jr, Davis PH, Leira EC, *et al.* Baseline NIH Stroke Scale score strongly predicts outcome after stroke: a report of the Trial of Org 10172 in Acute Stroke Treatment (TOAST). *Neurology.* 1999; 53: 126–31.
9 Hacke W, Donnan G, Fieschi C, *et al.*; ATLANTIS Trials Investigators; ECASS Trials Investigators; NINDS rt-PA Study Group Investigators. Association of outcome with early stroke treatment: pooled analysis of ATLANTIS, ECASS, and NINDS rt-PA stroke trials. *Lancet.* 2004; 363: 768–74.
10 Department of Health. *National Stroke Strategy.* London: DoH; 2007.
11 Dennis MS, Lewis SC, Warlow C; FOOD Trial Collaboration. Effect of timing and method of enteral tube feeding for dysphagic stroke patients (FOOD): a multicentre randomised controlled trial. *Lancet.* 2005; 365: 764–72.
12 de Vos R, Koster R, De Haan RJ, *et al.* In-hospital cardiopulmonary resuscitation: pre-arrest morbidity and outcome. *Arch Intern Med.* 1999; 159: 845–50.
13 British Medical Association. *Decisions Relating to Cardiopulmonary Resuscitation. A joint statement from the British Medical Association, the Resuscitation Council (UK) and the Royal College of Nursing.* London: BMA; 2007.
14 Department of Health. *Mental Capacity Act 2005.* London; Department of Health. Available at: www.justice.gov.uk

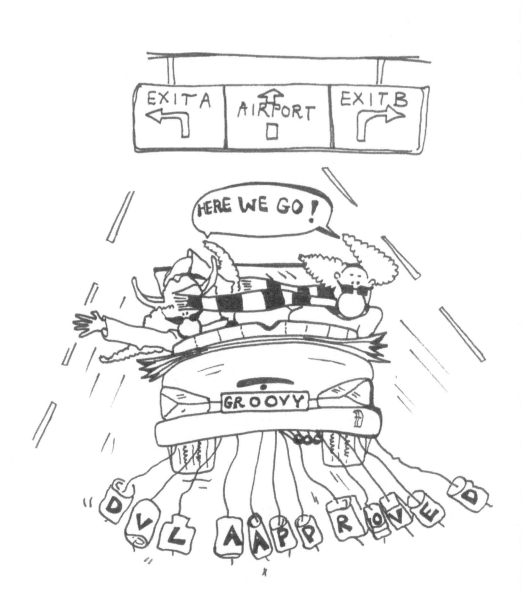

CHAPTER 10

Ethics of driving assessment in dementia: care, competence and communication

David Robinson and Desmond O'Neill

BACKGROUND

'We are bringing you to Dr O'Neill so that he can put you in a nursing home' would be a poor advertisement for a prospective patient with age-related disease about to attend a geriatric medicine clinic. The reasons for the unease generated by this phrase for both patients and practitioners are a useful guide to some of the issues related to ethics and driving. Both groups would be much happier with a formula along the lines of 'We are bringing you to Dr O'Neill to maximise your chances of staying at home. Of course, at some stage you may no longer be able to manage at home, and we may need to consider other options in the future.'

So what is the difference? The second formula:

➤ puts the needs and wishes of the patient to the fore, rather than those of the carer or society
➤ promotes the concept of geriatric medicine as enabling rather than disabling
➤ recognises a style of practice consistent with the World Health Organization (WHO)[1] and United Nations (UN)[2] guidelines which promotes due attention to prevention, health gain, health maintenance and palliation
➤ recognises the role of geriatric medicine in changing a societal mind-set towards disabling conditions of later life. Prior to the pioneering work of Marjorie Warren, the response of society was a prosthetic one, reinforcing

disability by premature admission to residential care. The key advance of geriatric medicine was to bring a diagnostic and therapeutic emphasis to the care of older people.

The contextual setting of the ethics of driving often seems to neglect the simple principles of care, competence and communication outlined above: 'care' in the sense of the appropriate focus of the practitioner – patient interaction; 'competence' in the sense of knowing not only the literature of assessment and remediation but also the extent of societal ageism; and 'communication' in the sense of understanding the skills needed to move from a primary focus on health gain to one of palliation. The primary ethos still appears to be 'We are bringing you to Dr O'Neill so that he can stop your driving' rather than 'We are bringing you to Dr O'Neill to maximise your changes of maintaining your mobility and transportation. Of course, at some stage you may no longer be able to drive, and we may need to consider other options in the future.' The literature in this area is a gloomy testament to the under-developed nature of the debate. The vast majority of the papers on Medline still focus on who should not drive, rather than considering the health implications of inadequate access to transport.

PUBLIC HEALTH ETHICS

The mis-emphasis probably arises from the processing of data by public health specialists whose primary role is the interpretation of accident analysis. An ethical imperative for such public health professionals is to become aware of the due proportionality of mobility and safety, and the importance of maintaining the balance in later life. This raises further issues with regard to how to ensure an input of gerontological training for public health professionals.

The challenge to geriatricians and gerontologists in relation to age-related disease and driving is to realign the context of mobility and risk. Some progress has already been made in this regard – the major impact of age-related disease is to curtail mobility.[3] A more measured sense of perspective has allowed a precious emphasis on risk to be reviewed – it is clear that older drivers are one of the safest groups of drivers on the road. A recent Organisation for Economic Co-operation and Development (OECD) report,[4] entitled *Ageing and Transport*, has re-emphasised that the main public health concerns of ageing and driving are twofold: first, reduced mobility and second, the hazard of increased frailty in an automotive and traffic environment that is not tailored to the needs of older people. Although older people as a group are the safest category of drivers on the road, the OECD pointed out the need for wider diffusion of assessment routines for clinicians dealing with drivers with known age-related disease.

DRIVING: A RIGHT AND A PRIVILEGE

Certain publications on driving assert that the possession of a driving license is a privilege, but in reality it is probably both a right and a privilege. All of our societies place a higher premium on mobility than on safety. If safety were the first priority, then the speed limit would be 20 miles per hour and car engines would be fitted with governors to prevent them exceeding this speed. The right to drive carries an implicit understanding of bearing a risk that is within certain societal norms. At all levels, older drivers as a group bear a risk that is low. A false argument is sometimes presented that their accident rate per mile travelled is high. This is false for two reasons: first, because they drive a lower mileage, their annual risk remains low; second, low mileage is intrinsically risky. If older and younger drivers are controlled for low mileage, their apparent increased risk disappears.[5,6]

These positive aspects of ageing are often under-appreciated, and the literature on ageing and mobility could benefit from a greater emphasis on the beneficial aspects of ageing. These include wisdom, strategic thinking and less risk taking. Even within the small proportion of crashes caused by drivers in this age group, the contribution of chronic disease to the crash risk is modest.[7] The safety record of older drivers in the face of these odds points to superior strategic and tactical skills. If skills were more widely applied, these qualities could enhance mobility and safety for all age groups.

ETHICAL HAZARDS IN CLINICAL SETTINGS

The ethical risks to practitioners in clinical practice are failure to consider driving as a part of their patient's functional status, a tendency to police rather than to enable, failure to refer appropriately for competence assessment, and inappropriate disclosure of information. The most striking example of failure to consider driving as a health-related issue comes from a study at a syncope clinic where referring physicians failed to alert many drivers (including lorry drivers) to stop driving until assessment and treatment were concluded.[8] There is some evidence that this agnosia is waning with time, although knowledge remains patchy.[9]

Against this background it is important to remember the primary duties and ethical responsibilities of the physician. First, to do no harm implies avoiding the damage to lifestyle, self-esteem and subsequently health that restrictions on driving may incur. For this reason we prefer to emphasise the empowering role of the physician – there is already much emphasis in the literature on limiting a patient's ability to drive. It is a physician's duty to promote the well-being of his or her patient, and it is important to remind ourselves that our role should be to enable patients to fulfil their potential, rather than to restrict it. Respecting patients' autonomy should enable us to allow patients to accept their own risk, but all too often they are not given this choice.

There has been a modest but significant increase in the literature on disease and driving. Some of this is original research and some represents a synthesis of prevailing wisdom. In many areas, physicians have more information than they did ten years ago. For example, with implantable cardiac defibrillators we know that the risk of crashes due to the defibrillator is low,[10] and we can predict those most at risk for syncope.[11] For cataracts, we know that older drivers with cataract experience a restriction in their driving ability and a decrease in their safety on the road.[12] We also know that surgical intervention can benefit older patients in terms of subjectively improved visual function and distance estimation while driving.[13] Such intervention translates to improved safety on the road.[14] For arthritis, while over half of patients affected report some difficulty driving,[15] we know not only that doctors fail to inquire about the impact of arthritis on mobility,[16] but also that a rehabilitative intervention programme can improve driving ease.[17] For diabetes, we have increasing evidence that the condition on its own has little or no effect on crash risk among older drivers without a history of crashes.[18]

ASSESSMENT

The assessment of patients' driving ability therefore requires certain minimum standards in order to assess fairly both ability to drive and risk to others. This involves remaining up to date with best practice, being aware of local legislation, and remaining cognisant of the massive impact that we have on a person's lifestyle. The competence required is that patients will have the most accurate assessment possible of their driving abilities. Schemata exist for the preliminary work in this area for physicians in primary care (e.g. the UK,[19] Australia,[20] Canada[21] and the USA[22]).

Just as not all chest pains arise from pulmonary emboli, clinicians need to have access to appropriate specialist expertise and technology to exclude the diagnosis in such cases. So, too, general physicians may need to invoke the assistance of a driving specialist centre, the components of which are medicine, occupational therapy, sometimes neuropsychology, and specialist driving assessors. A first effort may be made with a suitably trained occupational therapist – this profession is notable for upskilling in driving assessment in Australia, Canada and the USA. If this assessment is inconclusive, an on-road assessment is advisable. In the UK, such assessments are available from the Forum group of driver assessment centres. In the USA, the Association of Driver Rehabilitation Specialists (ADED; www.aded.net) can provide a list of suitably qualified driving assessors. It is important to emphasise to the patient that this test is not the driving test used for learner drivers, but rather it is an assessment designed to gain insight into the capabilities and difficulties of the driver.

THERAPEUTIC MANAGEMENT AND RISK ASSESSMENT

It is the placing of driving issues in an appropriate therapeutic context that is perhaps the most important task – non-clinician bioethicists thrive on the artificial heightening of potential conflict inherent in such situations. Rather than focusing on the difficult issue of patients who present late with impaired ability and insight, we need to recognise that the assessment of dementia provides the potential for a range of interventions, one of the most important of which is the establishment of a framework for advance planning in a progressive disease. Just as this is commonly recognised for such practical matters as enduring/lasting power of attorney in many jurisdictions, so too we need to start a process which encompasses an assessment and a commitment to maximising mobility, but also a process of awareness raising for the patient and their carers that the progression of the disease will inevitably result in a loss of driving capacity. This latter component has been termed a 'modified Ulysses contract' (after the hero who made his crew tie him to the mast of the ship on the condition that they did not heed his entreaties to be released when seduced by the song of the sirens).[23] Developing this process incorporates some new stances in dementia care, in particular disclosure of the diagnosis in at least general terms – the patient who drives needs to be told that they have a memory problem that is likely to progress and hamper their driving abilities. In general, carers are fearful of diagnosis disclosure but older people seem to want to be told if they have this illness. There is also evidence that such a process may facilitate driver cessation by enhancing a therapeutic dimension to disease diagnosis and advance planning.[24] It forms the basis of a useful patient and carer brochure from the Hartford Foundation, which is also available online.[25]

The commitment to maximising mobility must focus first on as accurate an assessment of the patient's driving abilities as possible, and second on exploring and planning alternative options for a future when driving is no longer possible. It is the promise of an attempt to maximise mobility that is the key to this transaction. If this is not a central component, we are faced with a dual ethical hazard. In the first instance, the therapeutic role of medicine is subjugated to an approach which inverts the standard of mobility-to-safety ratio to which we are all entitled. A further concern is that people with dementia may avoid assessment of the illness early in its course out of fear of unreasonable restriction of their mobility. As early diagnosis, treatment and management are considered to be desirable, this would be an unwelcome development.

The very act of highlighting the potential for compromised driving ability may have a therapeutic benefit, promoting increased vigilance on the part of the patient and carers about the fact that their social contract for driving privileges is not the same as that of the general public. Some support is given to this concept by the success of restricted licensing for people with medical illnesses in the state of Utah.[26] Although some of the effect might be due to the restrictions (avoidance of motorways and night-time driving), it is also possible that the very act of labelling these drivers may heighten their self-awareness.

The ethical component of risk is the onus on the physician to ensure that this has been assessed in the most accurate and professional manner possible. The greatest risk is to fail to refer the patient on for full assessment, perhaps on the basis that such expertise is geographically distant. Bear in mind that we would not let this deter us from arranging specialist neuroradiology for a suspected subdural haematoma or a ventilation/perfusion scan for a possible pulmonary embolus. We should apply similar criteria to the need for specialised assessments for impaired older drivers, particularly in view of the potential risk to other road users.

DISCLOSURE AND CONFIDENTIALITY

In general, the welfarist role of the physician extends to reminding the patient that most insurance companies require disclosure by the driver of 'illnesses relevant to driving' when they arise. Two issues arise. First, the medical advisers of the insurance companies may not make calculations of insurance rates (or continued insurance) on the basis of reason and evidence, but rather on ageist grounds and prejudice against disability. We may be unwittingly exposing the patient to this prejudice. The answer to this lies in continued advocacy by professional groups at a societal level as well as support by the physician in individual cases if the assessment supports preserved driving skills. A second issue is whether it is sufficient to recommend disclosure to someone who will not remember this advice. However, the physician's role is primarily to ensure safe mobility, and in general it is reasonable to assume that removal of insurance cover is a secondary matter in such cases. It is reasonable to share the disclosure of information with the carers.

The actual process of breaking confidentiality in the event of evidence of hazard to other members of the public is almost universally supported by most codes of medical practice. However, the question of to whom this should be reported poses some ethical challenges. The traditional route of reporting to driver licensing authorities (Division of Motor Vehicles in the USA, and Driver and Vehicle Licensing Authority in the UK) may have relatively little benefit, as removal of a driving licence is likely to have little impact on many drivers whose insight into deteriorating driving skills is poor. It is important that this disclosure has some likelihood of impact and results in the least traumatic removal of the compromised older driver from the road. In such instances, the family may be able to intervene in terms of disabling the car and providing alternative modes of transport. In our own experience, we rarely have to invoke official intervention, but find that a personal communication with a senior police officer in the patient's locality may result in a sensitive visit to the patient and cessation of driving.

Mandatory reporting presents a different ethical challenge. It is unlikely that it is of significant benefit and unless such benefit can be shown in future studies from mandatory reporting, the profession should resist the introduction of such schemes and fight against the maintenance of established schemes. For individual practitioners in jurisdictions where such regulations exist, a twin-track approach is probably necessary, involving professional advocacy with law makers and a considered approach as to whether disclosure is in the patient's best interests, on a case-by-case basis. If the physician is confident that the state or province has a mechanism for fair assessment and an enlightened approach to maintaining mobility, compliance is not difficult. If the assessment is cursory and aimed at unduly restricting mobility, physicians may be faced with a problem that is recognised with other laws, which may put patients' welfare at risk, and where professional obligations may require non-compliance with an unfair law.

CONCLUSION

The inclusion of driver assessment in clinical practice represents a new departure for the disciplines of applied ethics and ageing studies. It presents both challenges and opportunities, and involves not only clinicians but also public health professionals in ensuring that our practice represents a judicious balance between beneficence and non-maleficence, while at the same time keeping a firm perspective on the major issue, which is impaired mobility. The critical elements of care, competence and communication are the fundamentals of clinical practice which help to illuminate and clarify this equilibrium.

LEGAL POINTS

➤ In most countries, the legal obligation to disclose medical conditions that may impair driving lies with the driver.

➤ Professional codes of conduct usually allow for the breaking of medical confidentiality in the case of considered assessments of dangerous driving when such drivers will not cease driving.

➤ Courts in the UK have considered that doctors are bound to advise patients on conditions which may impair safe driving.[27]

REFERENCES

1 WHO. *Active Ageing: a policy framework.* Geneva: World Health Organization; 2002.

2 United Nations. *Report of the Second World Assembly on Ageing.* New York: United Nations; 2002.

3 Millar WJ. Older drivers – a complex public health issue. *Health Rep.* 1999; **11**(2): 59–71 (Eng); 67–82 (Fre).

4 OECD. *Ageing and Transport: mobility needs and safety issues.* Paris: Organisation for Economic Co-operation and Development; 2001.

5 Hakamies-Blomqvist L, Ukkonen T, O'Neill D. Driver ageing does not cause higher accident rates per mile. *Transport Res Part F, Traffic Psychol Behav.* 2002; 5: 271–4.

6 Langford J, Methorst R, Hakamies-Blomqvist L. Older drivers do not have a high crash risk – a replication of low mileage bias. *Accid Anal Prev.* 2006; **38**(3): 574–8.

7 McGwin G Jr, Sims RV, Pulley L, *et al.* Relations among chronic medical conditions, medications, and automobile crashes in the elderly: a population-based case-control study. *Am J Epidemiol.* 2000; **152**(5): 424–31.

8 MacMahon M, O'Neill D, Kenny RA. Syncope: driving advice is frequently overlooked. *Postgrad Med J.* 1996; **72**(851): 561–3.

9 Frampton A. Who can drive home from the emergency department? A questionnaire based study of emergency physicians' knowledge of DVLA guidelines. *Emerg Med.* 2003; **20**(6): 526–30.

10 Akiyama T, Powell JL, Mitchell LB, *et al.* The antiarrhythmics versus implantable defibrillators I. Resumption of driving after life-threatening ventricular tachyarrhythmia. *NEJM.* 2001; **345**(6): 391–7.

11 Bansch D, Brunn J, Castrucci M, *et al.* Syncope in patients with an implantable cardioverter-defibrillator: incidence, prediction and implications for driving restrictions. *J Am Coll Cardiol.* 1998; **31**(3): 608–15.

12 Owsley C, Stalvey B, Wells J, *et al.* Older drivers and cataract: driving habits and crash risk. *J Gerontol A Biol Sci Med Sci.* 1999; **54**(4): M203–11.

13 Monestam E, Wachmeister L. Impact of cataract surgery on the visual ability of the very old. *Am J Ophthalmol.* 2004; **137**(1): 145–55.

14 Wood JM, Carberry TP. Bilateral cataract surgery and driving performance. *Br J Ophthalmol.* 2006; **90**(10): 1277–80.

15 Cranney AB, Harrison A, Ruhland L, *et al.* Driving problems in patients with rheumatoid arthritis. *J Rheumatol.* 2005; **32**(12): 2337–42.

16 Thevenon A, Grimbert P, Dudenko P, *et al.* Polarthrite rhumatoïde et conduite automobile. *Rev Rhum Mal Osteoartic.* 1989; **56**: 101–3.

17 Jones JG, McCann J, Lassere MN. Driving and arthritis. *Br J Rheumatology.* 1991; **30**: 361–4.

18 McGwin G, Sims RV, Pulley L, *et al.* Diabetes and automobile crashes in the elderly. A population-based case-control study. *Diabetes Care.* 1999; **22**(2): 220–7.

19 DVLA. *At a Glance Guide to the Current Medical Standards of Fitness to Drive.* Swansea: Driver and Vehicle Licensing Authority; 2008.

20 Austroads. *Assessing fitness to drive.* Sydney: Austroads; 2003.

21 CMA. *Determining Medical Fitness to Operate Motor Vehicles.* 7th ed. Ottawa: Canadian Medical Association; 2006.

22 Wang CC, Kosinski CJ, Schwartzberg JG, *et al. Physician's Guide to Assessing and Counseling Older Drivers.* Washington, DC: National Highway Traffic Safety Administration; 2003.

23 Howe E. Improving treatments for patients who are elderly and have dementia. *J Clin Ethics*. 2000; **11**: 291–303.

24 Bahro M, Silber E, Box P, *et al.* Giving up driving in Alzheimer's disease: an integrative therapeutic approach. *Int J Geriatric Psychiatry*. 1995; **10**: 871–4.

25 Hartford Foundation. *At the Crossroads: a guide to Alzheimer's disease, dementia and driving*. Hartford, CT: Hartford Foundation; 2007.

26 Vernon DD, Diller EM, Cook LJ, *et al.* Evaluating the crash and citation rates of Utah drivers licensed with medical conditions, 1992–1996. *Accid Anal Prev*. 2002; **34**(2): 237–46.

27 Strawford G. Driving license revoked. *J MDU*. 1999; **15**: 18.

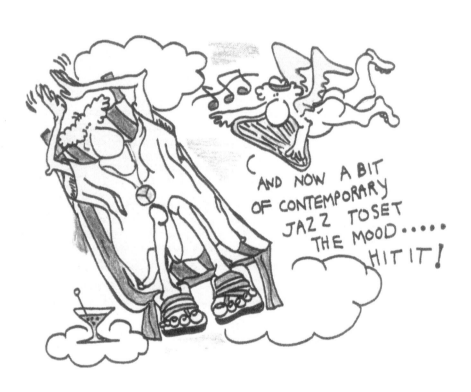

CHAPTER 11

Achieving a good death

Jim Eccles and Gurcharan S Rai

INTRODUCTION

There are between 50 000 and 100 000 'sudden' deaths in the UK each year due to natural causes, with the usual underlying pathologies being coronary artery disease, massive stroke and pulmonary embolism. Of the expected deaths many are foreseeable, with heart disease, cancer, stroke and respiratory disease being the major killers. A mercifully rapid final illness after enjoyment of an active life almost to the end is highly desirable, but in old age this is often not the outcome.

Traditionally, the term 'euthanasia', derived from the Greek words *eu* and *thanatos*, has simply meant 'a good death', but today it refers to the ending of life of a person who is suffering from advanced incurable illness, for his or her benefit, by another. What constitutes a 'good death'? The answer is three factors: the time to die, the place and the manner of death.

The time to die

The natural time to die is when the body can no longer sustain life, and this is usually in old age, since almost 80% of deaths in the UK occur in people over 65 years. Doctors who have the means to preserve organ function may need to ask themselves whether they are simply supporting vital physiological processes, or actually prolonging the process of dying.

The place to die

Most people, if asked, feel that they would prefer to die in their own homes, but the majority of us in the event die in institutions. Over half (54%) of all deaths occur in National Health Service (NHS) hospitals, 13% in private hospitals, residential care homes and nursing homes, and 4% in hospices. The remaining

29% occur in private households or elsewhere, such as in public places. To a varying extent, the doctor may have some influence over both where and how his or her patient dies. The Advance Care Planning guidance issued as part of the NHS End of Life Care Programme[1] emphasises the patient's right to choose where they wish to be cared for, at the end of life.

The way to die

There are many aspects of how we die, and here the doctor may have an important role. Three principles proposed by Jeffery and Millard[2] provide the doctor with tools to solve moral dilemmas at the end of life. These are as follows.

1 Treatment of patients must reflect the inherent dignity of every person irrespective of age, debility, dependence, race, colour or creed. The basis of the ancient Hippocratic oath is respect for the person as an individual in all aspects of medical and nursing management, including the period when withdrawal of treatment is being considered. The value of the person does not depend on whether treatment is useful or not.

2 Actions taken must reflect the needs of the patient where he or she is. Doctors' actions should not only display the highest standards of professional behaviour, but should also consider perceived burdens and benefits to the patient, their family, professional health carers and the community.

3 Decisions taken must value the person and accept human mortality. Although it is the doctor's duty to do no harm, it is not his or her duty to preserve life at all costs. When a medical treatment or intervention is no longer appropriate to sustain life, or the means used to sustain life are out of proportion to the life achieved, death should be accepted and allowed to take its course.

If the patient can make meaningful choices about the nature of such treatment options, then the patient's own views should be sought, especially if those choices involve subjective judgements about the 'quality' of the life that remains.

DILEMMAS FACED BY DOCTORS WHEN DEALING WITH DEATH
Should the doctor tell or not tell?

This question relates to both diagnosis and prognosis. According to the General Medical Council (GMC),[3] doctors should share with the patient whatever they need or want to know, especially in the context of treatment decisions. The GMC advises doctors not to make assumptions about the information which an individual patient might want or need. We may simply tell the patient of our suspicion that there is something serious going on until that suspicion has been confirmed. Otherwise we could unnecessarily alarm the patient by sharing a wide differential diagnosis, which may unreasonably remove hope at an early stage. However, although patients have a right to know, perhaps they also have a right not to know. We are all familiar with patients who seem to desist pointedly from asking anything which could lead to a disclosure of the diagnosis. This plea not to be told should be respected, although opportunities to ask questions should continue to be offered. Sometimes it is a close relative who requests that the truth be withheld – 'She's always been terrified of cancer, doctor, she'd simply give up if she knew.' Such requests are usually misguided, and most patients can come to terms with the reality much better once it has been brought out into the open. Furthermore, a web of deceit puts family relationships under a great strain. When the patient is dying, it is particularly appropriate that the patient should set the pace of the discussions about prognosis. One of the most difficult aspects of these discussions is the degree of uncertainty involved, but if we can share at least what we know, we can help our patients to make timely choices about their own palliative care.

Who should tell?

Ideally, this person should be a trusted and familiar doctor or nurse in the presence of someone who is particularly close to the patient. All too often it turns out to be a stranger in the outpatient clinic or in a hospital ward, and every effort should be made to avoid this.

Breaking bad news

Although they are not very strongly evidence based, here are a few guidelines for performing this unwelcome task in a kind and courteous way.

1 Do not strive for too much detachment – patients and their relatives seem to appreciate it if the doctor or nurse is affected emotionally.
2 Try not to kill all hope, or to give too precise a forecast of the duration of the illness. Offer a second opinion if one is wanted.
3 Sit down to indicate that you have time for discussion. Do not be afraid of eye contact, appropriate physical contact or silence. Describe your findings, the possible actions and the reasons for the prognosis.
4 Undertake to continue support and relieve symptoms. It is essential that the patient does not feel abandoned.

Consequent 'end-of-life decisions'

Patients may have conditions which severely limit both the duration and quantity of expected life, such as a disseminated malignancy, a gangrenous leg or severe cardiac failure. They may have conditions which limit the experience and quality of life, such as end-stage dementia or recurrent and severe stroke disease. In such situations it becomes reasonable to emphasise the relief of distressing symptoms and the preservation of dignity.

THE PATIENT IN THE COMMUNITY

Should a medical emergency arise in the care of a dying patient, general practitioners (GPs) need to think long and hard before sending the patient into hospital. If they decide to do so, then they need to make it clear to the receiving doctor that the primary reason for admission is to access more intense nursing support, or specialist advice, rather than 'heroic' intervention. This is an important time to consider the locally available alternative models of palliative care at home, and some out-of-hours primary care services are now involved in making these choices more accessible. In the case of patients living in nursing homes, it is important that any advance care plans include the consideration of locally available options for continuing palliative care in the home, if the patient wants to avoid further hospital admission. The Chief Medical Officer recommends influenza immunisation for older people, and although patients should be assessed for this in light of their individual prognosis, the impact on other vulnerable older people (such as fellow residents in a care home) of a failure to immunise should also be considered.

THE HOSPITAL PATIENT

Decisions about whether or not to subject patients to attempted cardiopulmonary resuscitation, or critical care support, should be taken in the context of their overall prognosis. In the case of patients receiving palliative care, it is particularly important to approach such decisions with sensitivity and tact. In hospital, the usual course is to record a resuscitation status in the notes. This is sensible, because in the event of a cardiac arrest there is no time to mull over the pros and cons of cardiopulmonary resuscitation. The decision is taken by the most senior doctor available,[4] after discussion with the rest of the team, the patient if he or she is able to participate in decision making, and the family in the case of a person who is incapacitated. It is not necessary to discuss futile interventions with a patient, but if it is thought that treatment decisions will depend on the anticipated result in terms of quality of life, then the patient should be consulted. The emphasis that is placed on recording the patient's resuscitation status should not prevent us from addressing those other treatment decisions which may be even more relevant to patients nearing the end of life, such as those concerned with nutritional support. A 'do not attempt resuscitation' (DNAR) decision does not imply that we are now only providing palliative rather than curative treatment; for instance, it should not automatically lead to the withholding of intravenous fluids or antibiotics.

ADVANCE CARE PLANNING

Some elderly people wish to declare in advance that, in the event of serious illness and incompetence to participate in decision making due to unconsciousness or confusion, they would not wish for particular life-supporting measures. These advance decisions to refuse treatment should ideally be drawn up in consultation with their GP, and other health professionals involved in their care. The Mental Capacity Act 2005 put advance decisions on a statutory footing. However, under the Act an advance decision will not apply to life-sustaining treatment unless it includes a statement that it should apply 'even if life is at risk' and the statement is signed, and witnessed.

Advance decisions present obvious practical difficulties. As a simple example, who will be aware of the decision if a person is rushed to hospital at night as an emergency? More fundamentally, it is impossible to envisage in advance every possible medical scenario that might arise. For these reasons, some people may choose to appoint an attorney to act on his or her behalf under a lasting power of attorney (LPA) but the attorney will only be able to make a healthcare decision once an individual becomes incapacitated (*see also* Chapter 8). The National Council for Palliative Care has produced guidance for health and social care professionals,[5] so that they will be able to assist patients to complete an advance decision, and it includes a model advance decision form.

THE ROLE OF CLOSE FRIENDS AND RELATIVES

It is obviously right for doctors to make themselves available to patients' families, and many complaints may arise from poor communication between health service staff and patients' relatives. In the case of infants, the parents have a decision-making capacity, within reasonable limits. In the case of adults, the immediate family does not, but the sensible doctor will listen attentively to their views. However, the ultimate responsibility for the decision is the doctor's. The motives of the relatives are in any case sometimes rather mixed. Those who demand that all possible life-saving measures should be taken may feel guilty after years of worry about whether they are neglecting an ailing relative. Those who suggest that it would be kinder to withdraw further aggressive treatment may be desperate to get their hands on the inheritance!

The Mental Capacity Act 2005 provides guidance on decision making on behalf of incompetent adults who require 'serious medical treatment':

1 consider if the decision can be delayed until the patient is capable of making the decision himself or herself, and if not

2 enquire if the patient has a valid and applicable advance decision

3 enquire if the patient has appointed an LPA for healthcare decisions

4 if there is no one appropriate to act as a 'natural advocate' for the patient,

request the appointment of an independent mental capacity advocate (IMCA)

5 where there is remaining disagreement about the patient's best interests, the decision should be referred to the Court of Protection.

EUTHANASIA

Definitions

➤ *Voluntary euthanasia*: the deliberate and intentional hastening of death at the request of the patient, who is seriously ill.

➤ *Involuntary euthanasia*: the ending of a person's life without seeking his or her opinion.

➤ *Non-voluntary euthanasia*: the ending of a person's life, for his or her own benefit, when that person cannot express or cannot possess views about whether he or she lives or dies.

➤ *Physician-assisted suicide*: the patient takes deliberately lethal medication by him or herself which has been prescribed or provided by the physician.

Euthanasia in the context of end-of-life care

The main decision confronting the doctor of a patient near the end of life is whether the aim should be palliation of symptoms or cure of the underlying cause. Most doctors subscribe to the traditional doctrine that good palliative care may involve gradually increasing the dosage of sedatives and analgesics with the aim of relieving suffering and distress, although this may have the unintended consequence of hastening the patient's death through depression of respiration, cough and movement (the so-called 'double effect'). The House of Lords Select Committee concluded in 1993 that it is proper to give doses of analgesic drugs and/or sedatives adequate to produce symptomatic relief, even if that action has the secondary consequence of shortening life. In such cases, it is the doctor's intent which is crucial. It is important to understand that increasing the dosage of pain-killing drugs, such as morphine, does not necessarily hasten death. Sometimes it is found that controlling the pain reduces the need for sedation and enhances the duration and quality of life.

If a patient has a colonic carcinoma with widespread metastases, that is now threatening to cause obstruction, a surgeon might perform a palliative bypass procedure, but no one would expect him or her to carry out a radical resection, on the grounds that it would be futile. In this situation, no one would use the term 'passive euthanasia'. If a patient with Down's syndrome was denied antibiotics for pneumonia, people might use that expression, although the most pressing question in such a case might be why a potentially life-prolonging treatment was withheld, and whether there was an element of discrimination. The term 'passive euthanasia' implies that decisions to withhold or withdraw life-prolonging treatment have been taken with the intention that the patient will die. Such decisions are specifically defined as being against the law in the UK in the case of incapacitated patients, according to the Mental Capacity Act 2005. Although some philosophers regard such withdrawals of treatment as 'passive euthanasia', the primary intention of the doctor is critical. If the doctor's intention is palliation and the medical intention of palliative care is the relief of distress, and treatment decisions may be based on a judgement of the value or futility of available treatment options, in the context of the patient's condition. An accurate assessment of the patient's mental and physical condition is therefore necessary, but there should be no attempt to judge the worth or futility of the patient's life, which is a matter for deeply personal and subjective consideration by the patient alone. Stopping treatment because a patient is dying, and stopping treatment because the doctor wants the patient to die, are not the same thing. It is therefore important that doctors record not only their palliative care treatment plans, but also the intention of those plans, in order to avoid misinterpretation of their motives.

The practice of active euthanasia, on the other hand, implies an intention to hasten the death of the patient on the basis of the presumed benefit of hastening death. Both intended euthanasia and physician-assisted suicide are strictly against the law in the UK.

The British Medical Association[6] has debated the issues at many national meetings, and in October 2007 the BMA:

➤ believes that the ongoing improvement in palliative care allows patients to die with dignity
➤ insists that physician-assisted suicide should not be made legal in the UK
➤ insists that voluntary euthanasia should not be made legal in the UK
➤ insists that non-voluntary euthanasia should not be made legal in the UK
➤ insists that if euthanasia were legalised, there should be a clear demarcation between those doctors who would be involved in it and those who would not.

Civilised society (respect for life)
  Assisted suicide (competent patient seeks help to commit suicide)
    Voluntary euthanasia (competent patient expresses wish to be put to death)
      Altruistic euthanasia (request for euthanasia for the benefit of others)
        Dutiful euthanasia (based on the social acceptance of a 'duty to die')
          Non-voluntary euthanasia (incompetent patient unable to express opinions)
            Involuntary euthanasia (social decision, patient's opinion not sought)
              Barbaric society (no respect for life)

BOX 11.1 The 'slippery slope' in end-of-life care.

One argument against euthanasia is that of the 'slippery slope' – for example, that there might be a gradual moral decline of society through unethical actions which become increasingly acceptable (*see* Box 11.1).

The Human Rights Act 1998 has been used on both sides of the debate surrounding euthanasia. It declares a right to life, but also states that people should not be subjected to inhuman or degrading treatment, and that they should be free from torture. The courts have not interpreted this as permitting the right of competent individuals to die by active euthanasia. This was demonstrated in the case of Mrs Pretty, who had a debilitating and terminal illness. She wanted her husband to be exempt from prosecution in the event that he assisted her in ending her life. The UK courts rejected this, and the decision was upheld in Europe.

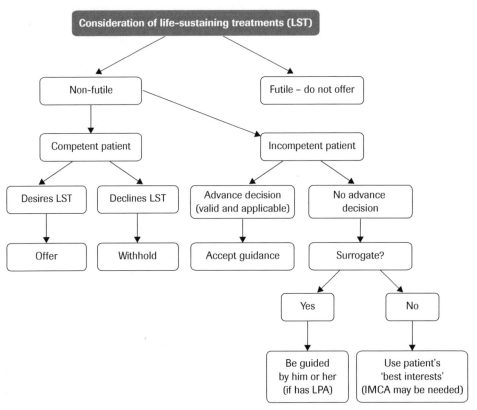

FIGURE 11.1 Consideration of life-sustaining treatments

The key question that doctors are expected to ask themselves in each case is therefore 'Is the treatment worthwhile or futile?' and not 'Is the patient's life worthwhile or futile?' If the decision depends on the perceived quality of a patient's life after treatment, then every effort should be made to understand that life as viewed from the patient's own, unique perspective (*see* Figure 11.1).

RELIGION

Although our society has become increasingly secular, for many people a good death will involve respect for their religious beliefs. Religion can offer some understanding of mortality. The ceremonies and rituals that surround dying can be a comfort both to patients and to their families. An understanding of religious beliefs is useful for comprehending attitudes to death, and an appreciation of these different customs is important for those involved in the care of dying patients.

Most religions promote the protection and care of those who are dying, and therefore forbid euthanasia. The monotheistic faiths, such as Christianity, Judaism and Islam, teach that life is sacred as it is given by God, and therefore ending a life is prohibited. While they teach that all life has a value, they also acknowledge that life need not be preserved at all costs. There is a recognition of the compassionate necessity to alleviate suffering and preserve dignity. As always, there is a spectrum of beliefs within these faiths. For example, the Orthodox Jewish tradition attaches much more importance to prolonging life than do other faiths. In Buddhism and Hinduism, there is a little more ambiguity because of the belief in reincarnation. Hastening the end of life would interfere with this process and go against the principle of *ahimsa* (doing no harm). However, there is a distinction between selfish reasons for ending life and spiritual or compassionate ones, such as the relieving of distress for relatives. These are great simplifications, but in general there is a consensus of opinion against euthanasia.

CASE HISTORIES

A number of case histories are given below, which illustrate some of the situations that may arise as death approaches. The patients are all elderly, representing the age group in which the large majority of deaths occur in the developed world. The real message behind these cases is that end-of-life decisions are often difficult, and there may be no clear-cut right or wrong answers. The patient's autonomy is paramount and the patient's views should always be respected, when the necessary mental capacity has been demonstrated. Even when mental capacity appears to be impaired, we should listen hard to our patients, in order to understand those preferences that can still be expressed.

CASE 11.1

Mr A, aged 82 years, was admitted with right lower lobe pneumonia. Two years previously he had a stroke and was profoundly dysarthric and unable to swallow solids or fluids without aspirating or choking. Two weeks ago, his wife had died but he had an elderly dog of which he was inordinately fond. His presumed aspiration pneumonia responded well to antibiotics, but he pulled out a nasogastric tube and refused a percutaneous endoscopic gastrostomy (PEG). He wrote several pathetic notes to the medical staff begging to be allowed home. It was felt that he was not truly depressed, but that death by dehydration and starvation alone in his cold and cheerless home would be a very sad fate. After discussion with his GP, and a careful assessment of his mental capacity, his request was acceded to, and he was doing well several months later.

Comments

1 The competent patient is always right.
2 The elderly thrive far better in their own homes.
3 Best interests are personal. (Two patients with identical medical conditions may have entirely different best interests.)

CASE 11.2

Mrs B, aged 80 years, was admitted via the Accident and Emergency department from her residential care home where she had sustained a number of falls. Two years previously she had been diagnosed as having severe dementia, and she was now agitated and aggressive, incontinent, and variably mobile with a frame and some assistance. On his ward round, the geriatrician recorded a DNAR order in her notes. The care staff from her home reviewed her, but felt unable to have her back, so attempts were made to find a nursing-home placement. One morning Mrs B choked and aspirated, and the house officer initiated intravenous antibiotics, despite which she died. Her son subsequently complained on the grounds that:

- the DNAR decision was unjustified
- it should have been discussed with him
- it may have been made simply because the hospital needed the bed (!).

Comment

- A DNAR decision does not necessarily involve other non-treatment decisions unless specified.
- Even if a DNAR decision is made on the grounds of medical futility, it is good practice to keep the family closely informed if the patient has lost the mental capacity to participate in discussion.

CASE 11.3

Mrs C, aged 78 years, who was residing in a nursing home due to multiple strokes, was sent into hospital by a visiting GP because she had ceased to eat or drink. She was profoundly dehydrated, severely dysphagic, had an indwelling catheter, and the electrolytes showed a sodium level of 183 mmol/l and a urea level of 48.9 mmol/l. She received intravenous rehydration, as the on-call team felt that this was the GP's intention and the consultant doing the 'post-take ward round' decided to send her back to the familiar surroundings of the nursing home. However, during an acrimonious interview her six sons and daughters insisted that their mother was mentally intact, valued her life, and would wish for PEG feeding, a request to which the consultant reluctantly acceded.

Comment
1 You are treating the patient, not the family, but you should gracefully accept that they often know the patient better than you do.
2 The sight of a loved one in a physically vulnerable state may trigger an understandable, but highly protective response.
3 Nutritional support in dysphagic stroke survivors is the most sensitive issue in the management of stroke patients. Current guidance is to feed with a nasogastric tube, and later convert to PEG feeding if dysphagia persists (in order to maintain nutrition rather than to guarantee protection of the airway), except in cases where the prognostic indicators are so bad that prolongation of life is contrary to the patient's best interests.
4 Try to encourage the family to consider the issue in context of the overall prognosis.
5 If discussion with the family becomes difficult, an early offer of a second opinion may reassure them that we are considering all aspects of the case.
6 If the patient recovers, try to establish an agreed care plan which incorporates a strategy for managing similar crises in the future.

CASE 11.4

Mr D, aged 78 years, was sent into hospital with rapidly increasing breathlessness, and was found to be cachectic and to have a large pleural effusion with a 'white-out' on the X-ray. The fluid was bloodstained, but no malignant cells were found, so the respiratory physician was contacted. He suggested further aspiration for cytology and, if the result was still negative, a pleural biopsy after stopping the warfarin that Mr D was still taking for previous pulmonary emboli. This procedure was performed a week later, by which time Mr D had become progressively weaker, and he died shortly thereafter.

Comment

- The consideration of what investigations may be in the patient's best interests depends on doctors having clear goals in terms of possible benefits, and a clear understanding of the risks involved.
- These should be shared with the patient (if mentally competent) or those people who are close to the patient.
- Our discussions need to include an honest expression of any diagnostic or therapeutic uncertainty.

SUMMARY OF END-OF-LIFE DECISIONS

1 Will further investigation clarify the overall management?
2 Information should be shared with the patient and/or the family.
3 Resuscitation decisions should be taken in context of the overall prognosis.
4 Is the aim of treatment a cure of underlying pathology, or primarily palliative?
5 A distinction between the withdrawal of active treatment as part of palliative care, and the intentional ending of human life, is supported by both the UK law and medical profession (BMA).

REFERENCES

1 Department of Health. *NHS End of Life Care Programme Advance Care Planning: a guide for health and social care staff.* London: Department of Health; 2008. Available at: www.endoflifecareforadults.nhs.uk/eolc/eolcpub.htm (accessed 15 April 2009).
2 Jeffery P, Millard PH. An ethical framework for clinical decision-making at the end of life. *J R Soc Med.* 1997; 90: 504–6.
3 General Medical Council. *Consent: patients and doctors working together.* London: GMC; 2008. Available at: www.gmc-uk.org/guidance/ethical_guidance/consent_guidance/contents.asp (accessed 15 April 2009).
4 British Medical Association. *Decisions Relating to Cardiopulmonary Resuscitation.* London: BMA; 2007. Available at: www.bma.org.uk/ap.nsf (accessed 15 April 2009).
5 National Council for Palliative Care. *Advance Decisions to Refuse Treatment: a guide for health and social care professionals.* London: National Council for Palliative Care; 2008. Available at: www.adrtnhs.co.uk/
6 British Medical Association. *End-of-life Decisions: BMA views.* London: BMA; 2007. Available at: www.bma.org.uk/ap.nsf (accessed 15 April 2009).

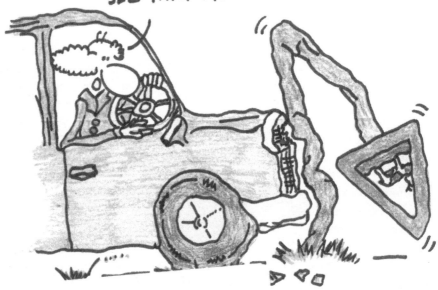

CHAPTER 12

Ethical issues in dementia

Gurcharan S Rai and Jim Eccles

INTRODUCTION

Dementia is a disease that shows increasing incidence with age. While the prevalence is about 5% in the elderly over 65 years of age, it reaches nearly 20% in those over 80 years. In clinical practice it is important to differentiate not only between acute confusional states and dementia, but also between the various types of dementia as new treatments for Alzheimer's disease become available.

Ethical issues arising in the management of dementia vary with progression of the disease. In the early stages, issues may range from questions of consent, to informing the patient that he or she has a dementing illness, to decision-making capacity. In the later stages, the issues revolve around appropriate levels of care, decisions about resuscitation and end-of-life issues, financial/legal arrangements and restraining. Although there is no cure for dementia, new therapies are being developed to improve function and/or slow down the progression of disease. The recent introduction of anticholinesterase inhibitors such as donepezil, rivastigmine and gallantamine has raised the ethical issue of rationing/postcode prescribing.

Over time, alteration in a patient's cognitive state may lead to a change in the doctor–patient relationship. It is not uncommon to note that a physician, after having assessed the patient, talks to the carer as if the patient were not in the room, thus ignoring the patient's feelings. It is important for us as professionals to recognise that loss of cognitive function does not mean total loss of emotions and human values. At the very least, the physician should ensure that the patient is seen on his or her own before any discussion takes place between the doctor and the carer, and any discussion that takes place should involve the patient.

ETHICAL ISSUES IN THE EARLY STAGES OF DEMENTIA

In the early stages, patients with dementia have the capacity to undertake decisions with regard to their treatment (i.e. they can choose to accept or refuse), and therefore should not be treated any differently from other patients but instead be allowed to exercise that choice. Denying choice compromises independence and dignity. The National Institute for Health and Clinical Excellence (NICE) recommends that while a person with dementia has capacity, there should be full discussion with him or her and his or her carers on the use of:

➤ advance statements on what action should be taken if the person loses the capacity to make decisions
➤ advance decisions to refuse treatment
➤ lasting power of attorney
➤ a preferred place of care.

Informing the patient about the diagnosis

It is argued by some that because dementia is a progressive disease with no available curative treatment, some patients will be unable to accept the diagnosis, and as a result may suffer psychological distress with a subsequent reduction in hope and motivation. Although it is true that, in practice, some patients find it difficult to accept a diagnosis with a poor prognosis (e.g. they switch off during discussion), it should be possible to discuss the diagnosis sympathetically, providing support to the patient over two or more sessions. Basic principles require that we as physicians should be honest and tell the patient the truth so that they can exercise their moral and ethical right to decide, while they are still competent, whether they wish to accept or reject treatment or investigations should they become incompetent. This may also lead to patients accepting the involvement of support groups or help from psychologists and community psychiatric nurses. This in turn helps through discussion to overcome psychological reactions of fear, depression and anger. In addition, patients may decide to seek guidance about advance refusals (advance directives). If there is a language barrier, the doctor should consider using independent interpreters or using written information in the preferred language and/or an accessible format.

In some cases, family members may insist that a patient should not be informed of the diagnosis. Under these circumstances it is important to clarify that a competent individual has the moral and legal right to know the diagnosis and make decisions about their future care, which also includes treatment.

Informing family/carers about the diagnosis

Family members may not only ask for the diagnosis to be kept from the patient, but may also ask for the diagnosis to be given to them before it is given to the patient. In the latter situation it is important to inform the family that doctors cannot, either in law or ethically, give information to a third party without the consent and agreement of a competent adult (i.e. the patient). In fact, a competent patient can ask a doctor not to talk to a particular family member, and if this happens, doctors must act in accordance with the patient's wishes. Of course in the late stages of dementia, when the patient is unlikely to have the capacity to give consent, the doctor should talk to the family. Sharing information with the family and carer involved in providing support and care to the patient will not only help the doctor to obtain insight into the patient's past wishes, but will also ensure that appropriate care is organised in the best interests of the patient.

Issues surrounding genetics

Recent developments in genetics have identified mutations that predispose to Alzheimer's disease on chromosomes 21, 19, 14 and 1. The gene located on chromosome 21, an autosomal-dominant gene, was the first to be discovered in groups of families in whom the onset of dementia started at below the age of 65 years. This gene results in the production of a precursor protein B-amyloid around plaques. The genetic abnormality on chromosome 19, the second to be discovered, represents a risk factor for individuals over the age of 60 years. The allele associated with increased risk is e4. The third abnormal gene, located on chromosome 14 (an autosomal-dominant gene), is responsible for 70–80% of familial cases. The fourth gene locus, on chromosome 1, relates to an early onset of familial dementia. Although chromosome 1 is a dominant gene, at least two examples of probable incomplete penetrance have been identified. The three disease genes responsible for familial Alzheimer's dementia (chromosomes 21, 14 and 1) account for fewer than 5% of all cases. Therefore in the majority of patients with Alzheimer's dementia, it is a polygenic multifactorial disorder in which some gene effects may be found, but environmental and other modulatory factors may be of central importance.

Although some physicians and relatives may suggest or demand screening for families, particularly for those with familial Alzheimer's disease, the majority reject it on the grounds that there is no preventative or protective treatment currently available, and that it has the additional disadvantage of causing psychological trauma for the individual and their family. The Nuffield Council on Bioethics has advised against the introduction of genetic testing in disorders/ diseases with multiple causes, and thus this applies to most if not all older patients with Alzheimer's disease. If a doctor agrees to the demand for genetic testing from a member of the family of a patient with familial Alzheimer's disease, counselling before and after testing is regarded as essential in line with recent NICE guidance.

Ethical issues surrounding new treatment

At present there are four drugs available for use in patients with Alzheimer's disease, namely donepezil (a piperidine-based reversible inhibitor of acetylcholinesterase), rivastigmine (a centrally selective inhibitor of acetylcholinesterase), gallantamine (a competitive acetylcholinesterase inhibitor) and memantine (a voltage-dependent, moderate-affinity non-competitive NMDA-receptor antagonist). Donepezil, rivastigmine and gallantamine are recommended for patients with moderate severity only (MMSE 10–20). Memantine is no longer recommended for patients in the later stages of the disease, except as part of well-designed clinical study. In line with NICE guidelines, only specialists in the care of patients with dementia (i.e. psychiatrists, neurologists and physicians specialising in care of the elderly) are allowed to prescribe with regular review at six months using the Mini-Mental State Examination (MMSE) score, global, functional and behavioural assessments. Of course, MMSE may not be appropriate as a tool for assessment for those from different ethnic groups and patients with disabilities. In these patients it is important to consider using alternative tests such as the Cambridge Cognitive Examination (CAMCOG), Modified Cambridge Examination for Mental Disorders of the Elderly (CAMDEX), Dementia Questionnaire for Mentally Retarded Persons (DMR) or Dementia Scale for Down's Syndrome (DSS). None of these drugs is curative, and not all patients with Alzheimer's disease show a response to them.

The introduction of these drugs has not met with universal enthusiasm from health authorities, and they may question the value of this treatment, on the grounds of cost effectiveness. The concept of cost effectiveness, as analysed by NICE, has been closely associated with their use of the quality-adjusted life year (QALY), which has been the subject of a lively debate in the ethics literature. The use of the QALY by NICE, in order to calculate the effectiveness of new treatments, has been challenged on the grounds that physicians cannot objectively judge the quality of an individual life, since the only person qualified to make that judgement is the person living it.

Although it is reasonable not to offer treatment that is deemed futile, it is ethically wrong – and may soon be illegal – to deny treatment on the grounds of cost alone, if that treatment has been shown to be of benefit. The NICE guidance on prescribing in dementia has recently been subjected to a judicial review, and it is important that any rationing on the grounds of cost effectiveness is open to both legal and political scrutiny.

The other ethical issue in relation to prescribing of anti-dementia drugs is that of consent. In UK law, an adult is presumed to have the capacity to make decisions and to act upon those decisions. Therefore it follows that before an anti-dementia drug can be prescribed, a doctor must obtain the patient's consent. However, significant numbers of patients with dementia are incapable of giving consent, and if the ethical guidelines on consent to treatment are strictly adhered to, many of these patients would be wrongly deprived of treatment from which they could benefit. Therefore it is accepted practice that if patients cannot give consent to medical treatment, the doctor should act in the patient's best interest after full consideration of the benefits and unwanted effects of the treatment, and after full consultation with the family/carers who know the patient best.

Issues surrounding patients' liberty to drive

Dementia can lead not only to changes in memory but also to impairment of judgement, visuospatial difficulties and inattentiveness. All of these changes can affect driving, and there is evidence that a diagnosis of dementia is associated with an increased risk of accidents. Patients with Alzheimer's dementia are five times more likely to have a car accident than their age-matched health controls. This raises the following questions:

1 what advice should doctors give to patients with dementia?
2 what should happen if patients continue to drive against their doctor's wishes?
3 what is the law regarding fitness to drive?

What advice should doctors give to patients with dementia?

The answer to this question should be based on a full assessment of the patient, since not all patients with a diagnosis of dementia become unfit to drive at the time when the diagnosis is made. In the early stages there may not be any gross difficulties with judgement, visual perception, visuospatial discrimination or attention. Under these circumstances, patients can be advised that they may continue to drive until difficulties start to arise. However, if the patient admits to difficulties, a carer reports difficulties or the patient has a moderate degree of dementia, then that patient should be advised not to drive until a full assessment has been made. This may involve psychometric assessment by a psychologist and assessment by driver licensing authorities (such as the Driver and Vehicle Licensing Authority (DVLA) in the UK) to determine their medical fitness to hold a licence. The initial assessment by the DVLA consists of a medical enquiry about the patient addressed to his or her general practitioner (GP) regarding episodes of confusion or memory problems. In addition, they may ask for reports from consultant psychiatrists or an independent medical assessment and psychometric report. If doubt remains after this assessment, a full assessment may take place at a recognised Disabled Driver Assessment Unit, where physical and psychometric assessments are undertaken. If doubt about the person's ability to drive still persists, they may be asked to take a full driving test. Finally, it is important to note that simple cognitive tests such as the MMSE are very poor predictors of driving ability.

What should happen if patients continue to drive against their doctor's wishes?

It is important for us, as doctors, first to remember that we have a legal duty to respect the confidence of a patient, and second to consider not only the right of a person with dementia to maintain their personal freedom, but the right of everyone to be safe. Although reporting of suspected medical unfitness to drive raises an important ethical dilemma about confidentiality, most physicians now accept that the principle of confidentiality is partly or wholly balanced by a 'common good' principle for the protection of third parties. In the UK, the doctor should therefore inform the DVLA in Swansea directly on failure to persuade the patient to do this himself or herself, and when the doctor has grounds to suspect that the patient is putting himself or herself or others at risk.

What is the law regarding fitness to drive?

In the UK, the Road Traffic Act 1988 and the Motor Vehicles (Driver Licences) Regulations 1996 define severe mental disorder as a relevant disability for licensing, and this includes dementia. The person is obliged by law to inform the DVLA about his or her condition. If a patient refuses to do this despite advice from their doctor and family, the doctor can inform the DVLA directly after first informing the patient of this decision.

ETHICAL PROBLEMS ASSOCIATED WITH THE LATE STAGES OF DEMENTIA

As the disease progresses, patients become increasingly less able to make decisions. However, this does not imply incompetence. Although they may not understand the benefits and risks of medical intervention, they may still be able to understand their finances or home circumstances. Therefore it is essential that competence is assessed in the area in question.

Treatment of acute illness, including decisions about resuscitation

As the disease progresses, patients become mentally incompetent and therefore unable to make decisions about treatment. Under these circumstances one should consider the following three steps under the Mental Capacity Act 2005:

1 can the decision be delayed until the patient is capable of making the decision himself or herself? If answer is 'yes', then decision should be delayed; if not, then ask
2 if the patient has appointed a lasting power of attorney for personal and welfare decisions, or made a valid advance decision
3 if the answer to 2 is 'no', then the patient's best interest should be treated using the checklist (*see* Table 12.1).

TABLE 12.1 Checklist for determining the patient's best interests

Factors to be taken into account when making a 'best interests' assessment

- Identifying things that an individual would take into account if acting for him/herself

- Patient's past and present expressed wishes

- Patient's beliefs and values

- Views of family, friends, carers, GP – ask them what patient would have wanted

- Views of independent mental capacity advocate, if patient has no family or friends

In an emergency where formal capacity assessment is not possible, immediate treatment can be administered on the basis of assumed consent in a co-operating patient or in their best interest until the patient's condition has been stabilised, at which stage best interest assessment can be performed.

In reality, the clinical decision-making process may involve looking at the benefits as well as the risks, burdens and side-effects of treatment, and the patient's quality of life. Since quality of life is difficult to assess, it becomes increasingly necessary to make a judgement based on the severity and prognosis of the disease. If the patient is clearly nearing the end of life, it becomes both reasonable and acceptable not to attempt any futile treatment which could offer the false hope of artificially prolonging that life. Symptomatic treatments such as antipyretics for fever, mouth care, bowel care to prevent constipation, bladder care to prevent retention of urine, and skin care to prevent pressure sores all become increasingly important. As death becomes imminent, the priorities are symptom relief and personal dignity. In this situation, cardiopulmonary resuscitation should not be attempted, as it would not be an appropriate part of such a palliative care plan. Quite apart from being futile, attempts to revive a patient at such a late stage would also deprive both the patient and family of privacy and dignity at the end of a long illness.

Percutaneous endoscopic gastrostomy feeding

CASE 12.1

An 85-year-old woman who has severe Alzheimer's disease is admitted to hospital from a nursing home with right lower lobe pneumonia. Assessment by a speech and language therapist revealed poor swallowing on admission to hospital. Nurses start her on nasogastric feeding. During the next seven days the patient pulls out the nasogastric tube on six occasions. After the seven days, when her clinical features of pneumonia have improved, the question of percutaneous endoscopic gastrostomy (PEG) is raised. The speech and language therapist feels that the patient is unlikely to pull out her PEG as it does not normally cause discomfort.

Swallowing problems are not uncommon in patients with dementia with the progression of disease, and particularly at times of acute illness. In some the ability to swallow returns, while in others the swallowing difficulties remain, making oral intake unsafe. At this stage PEG may be considered and discussed as a long-term option between the members of the multi-disciplinary team and the family. Often the question of whether it is appropriate to place a PEG tube in a severely demented patient will be asked.

This dilemma is not uncommonly encountered by doctors who are caring for older people. In decision making, the doctor should consider the following.

➤ The benefits and risks associated with PEG in this group of patients. One large influential review failed to find any evidence that tube feeding patients with advanced dementia prolongs survival, prevents aspiration pneumonia, reduces the risk of pressure sores or improves physical function and comfort. In addition, PEG is associated with local irritation, which can lead to potentially fatal complications, such as infection and haemorrhage.

➤ The benefits and risks associated with PEG in the patient concerned. Co-morbidity in an individual increases the risk of complications and mortality.

➤ Whether the patient has left instructions in the form of a valid and applicable advance decision. Enquiry should also be made as to whether the patient has appointed an attorney, using the lasting powers of attorney, to cover medical treatment.

If the patient has not made an advance refusal or appointed an attorney to decide about medical treatment, then the decision should be made in the patient's best interests, using the assessment recommended by the Mental Capacity Act 2005, including the following.

➤ Discussion of the benefits and risks of PEG feeding with family, carers and staff involved in caring for the patient. An independent mental capacity advocate (IMCA) should be appointed if there are no suitable relatives or close friends to consult.

➤ Assessment of the patient's present behaviour. Is the patient trying to indicate that he or she does not wish to be fed, by pulling out nasogastric tubes repeatedly, or by declining to take food orally when it is offered? Alternatively, does the patient demonstrate signs of hunger, and a desire to try foods that may be deemed as unsuitable due to swallowing difficulties?

In some patients with dementia, dysphagia may not be due to the dementia itself, but may be the result of another physical condition. Under those circumstances it would be more appropriate to consider PEG feeding. However, if the decline in nutritional intake is due to the dementia itself, then the disease has reached a very advanced stage, and a more palliative approach to care may be indicated. The recent NICE–SCIE guidance recommends that tube feeding is not usually appropriate for patients with severe dementia who are nearing the end of life.

Use of physical and chemical restraints

Personality and behavioural changes are common with progression of the disease process. Aberrant behaviour with or without wandering, particularly in the presence of an acute illness, may become a major problem for the patient's carer/family as well as for professionals who are providing help and care for those affected by the disease. Although it would be wrong to restrain someone physically (and in the UK, it is against the law) or chemically just for the benefit of carers or hospital staff, it should be considered where it is in the best interest of the patient. Section 6 of the Mental Capacity Act, which defines 'restraint' as the use or threat of force where an incapacitated person resists, permits use of restraint if the person using it believes it is justifiable, because it is both necessary to prevent harm to the incapacitated person, and is proportionate to the likelihood and seriousness of the harm. One should also include the caregiver's views about any possible restraint in the decision-making process. The proposed ethical guidelines devised by the Ethics and Humanities Subcommittee of the American Academy of Neurology include the following:

1   restraints should be ordered when they contribute to the safety of the patient or others and are not simply a convenience for the staff
2   restraints should not be ordered as a substitute for careful evaluation and surveillance of the patient, as appropriate for good medical practice
3   the perceived need for restraints should trigger medical assessment and investigation of the precise reason for them, intended to correct the underlying medical or psychological problem
4   if a proxy decision maker is known, restraints should be ordered after full discussion of the risks and benefits. However, in an acute situation doctors should act in the best interest of the patient
5   when they are indicated, pharmacological agents should be used at the lowest dose possible
6   all restraints should be reassessed frequently so that they may be in effect for the shortest duration necessary to achieve their goals.

Use of monitoring equipment

Assistive technology continues to develop not only in order to enable independence for the elderly but also for the purpose of monitoring the well-being of an individual. Video and electronic tags are now widely available and are being employed by some institutions and private homes for monitoring elderly patients with dementia, who have a tendency to wander and a predisposition to fall. There is no doubt that the use of such equipment raises issues such as freedom/liberty, and it is therefore important that any decision to use them takes into account such important issues and places the individual older person at the centre of the decision-making process. The final decision should be based on the principle of 'best interest' of the older person, and not on the interest of the staff/carer or the home itself.

Law and financial handling capacity of patients with dementia

As dementia progresses, patients become increasingly less able to handle their financial affairs. In the early stages, an individual can ask another person to help collect a pension or pay bills on the odd occasion. However, for permanent arrangements the patient with dementia who has the capacity to understand and make decisions should be advised to make an enduring power of attorney.

Enduring power of attorney was introduced in England and Wales in 1985 to cover financial matters but not decisions on medical treatment or non-financial personal arrangements. The Mental Capacity Act 2005 has replaced it with the lasting power of attorney (LPA), which covers property and financial affairs as well as personal welfare covering social and medical care. To be effective, an LPA will have to be registered with the Office of the Public Guardian (OPG).

In financial matters, LPA gives 'general' authority to carry out all transactions on behalf of the individual, or specific authority. This gives the person authority to sign cheques or withdraw money from the bank.

When there is no LPA, the Court of Protection can be asked to appoint a deputy who will be able to take decisions on financial matters as authorised by the Court. Although the deputy can also be given authority to act on social and health matters, he or she will not have authority to refuse consent to life-sustaining treatment.

What about those who neglect themselves at home because of dementia but refuse to accept help?

In the late stages of dementia, personal neglect is not only common but often denied by the patient. Commonly this information becomes available when a person is admitted to hospital with an acute illness. A dilemma arises, with conflict between autonomy and beneficence, when the patient recovers from the physical illness and insists on going home. The individual's wishes (patient's autonomy) must be respected. Actions must be taken to reduce or minimise neglect as far as possible through discussion with the patient, their family/carers and all of the agencies involved in providing community services. If this is not possible, and the patient refuses to accept help or to leave home to go into a safer environment, and from assessment it is clear that the patient is unable to understand the risks of going home, then a decision should be taken in the patient's best interests. Even then, the Mental Capacity Act 2005 encourages us to consider the patient's wishes, and to choose the 'least restrictive option'. In the UK, 'guardianship' under the Mental Health Act 1983 can be exercised in order to ensure the welfare of the patient and the protection of others. This will allow the patient to be moved to a safer environment. To enforce this section, the signatures of two registered practitioners (one of whom should be a mental health specialist) are required.

The other sections of the Mental Health Act can also be used to detain patients with dementia. For example, under Section 4 a person can be admitted as an emergency if the relatives and social workers cannot cope with the patient's behaviour. The period of detention under the section is a maximum of 72 hours, but this can be changed to 28 days by seeking a specialist opinion.

Section 47 of the National Assistance Act 1948 can also be used to admit a person to hospital who is unable to care for himself or herself at home, is not receiving care at home, is suffering from a grave chronic disease or living in unsanitary conditions. This Act does not allow treatment to be given against the patient's wishes. The other drawback is that, unlike the Mental Health Act 1983, it does not provide safeguards for the person with respect to review procedures.

The recently revised Mental Health Act 2007 has amended the Mental Capacity Act, to include new safeguards to prevent the casual 'deprivation of liberty' in the care of people with impaired mental capacity. These new safeguards, which were implemented on 1 April 2009, will have a significant impact on the arrangements for the long-term care of such patients, and may also apply in the case of patients who need to be restrained while in hospital. They will require that a series of formal assessments of mental health, capacity and best interests are undertaken before the deprivation of liberty can be authorised. Although the Mental Health Act 2007 has not resulted in Section 47 of the National Assistance Act being repealed, it is clear that in cases where the new 'deprivation of liberty' safeguards are already in operation, they will take precedence. According to the wording of the Mental Health Act 2007, there would appear to be no reason why the new safeguards will not apply following an admission under Section 47, but this may ultimately need to be clarified by case law.

Abuse of the elderly with dementia

Mental impairment makes the elderly vulnerable to abuse, which may take the form of physical, mental and financial abuse as well as deprivation of nutrition, help in activities of daily living and prescribed drugs. Recognition of abuse can be difficult because physical changes may mimic the changes of ageing and the elderly person may be unwilling or unable to admit to abuse. Action against suspected abuse in an institution may be possible through statutory bodies that visit institutions and action against individuals who ill-treat or neglect a person who lacks capacity is possible using the Mental Capacity Act 2005, which has introduced this as a criminal offence that carries a penalty of imprisonment for a term of up to five years.

In the case of a person who is being abused and still has capacity, it is difficult to take action against a relative/carer who is suspected of abuse if the elderly person is unwilling or unable to co-operate. This raises the important ethical issue of whether action should be taken against the wishes of an elderly person in order to protect them. Unfortunately, there is no law that allows professionals to make the elderly Wards of Court, as is the case with children. Therefore we have no option but to work closely with all of the professionals involved in providing care for the older person. This also includes relatives, who unfortunately may themselves be the abusers of the elderly patient. It is hoped that vigilant and consistent contact will reduce the likelihood of abuse. To help with this process, local health authorities and social services have drawn up guidelines for staff to follow.

KEY POINTS

- In the early stages, patients with dementia have the full capacity to undertake decision making with regard to their treatment, and therefore should not be treated differently from other patients.
- Basic principles require the physician to tell the patient that he or she has dementia.
- Since there are no available preventative or therapeutic agents that can cure dementia, it is not yet necessary to carry out genetic testing to establish whether a family member has the relevant gene(s).
- Any new effective treatment that is developed should be available for patients, and no one should be denied treatment solely on the grounds of cost. Any rationing should be open to public scrutiny.
- Patients with obvious impairment of judgement or visuospatial difficulties should be asked to stop driving. If they fail to take this advice, they should be reported to the DVLA, even if it means breaking the rule about patient confidentiality.
- In the late stages of disease, doctors may have to make decisions about which treatment is best for the individual. Assessment of best interests should be performed in line with the Mental Capacity Act 2005.

- In end-stage dementia, artificial tube feeding is not usually appropriate, and palliative care should be available when required.
- Restraint should only be used if it contributes to the safety of the patient or others, and should not be used for the convenience of staff.
- In the early stages of dementia, patients should be encouraged to consider appointing an LPA, and making a valid advance decision.
- Patients who neglect themselves may still need to be admitted to hospital under Section 47 of the National Assistance Act, or moved into a residential home using guardianship under the Mental Health Act 1983.
- New safeguards to prevent the deprivation of liberty will be widely applicable to the care of patients with impaired mental capacity.

FURTHER READING

American Academy of Neurology, Ethics and Humanities Subcommittee. Ethical issues in the management of the demented patient. *Neurology.* 1996; 46: 1180–3.

Department of Health. *Reference Guide to the Mental Health Act 1983.* London: DoH; 2008. Available at: www.mhact.csip.org.uk/news/latest-news/reference-guide.html (accessed 15 April 2009).

Department for Constitutional Affairs. *Mental Capacity Act 2005 Code of Practice.* London: DCA; 2007. Available at: www.dca.gov.uk/menincap/legis.htm#codeofpractice (accessed 15 April 2009).

Finucane TE, Christmas C, Travis K. Tube feeding in patients with advanced dementia: a review of the evidence. *JAMA.* 1999; 282: 1365–70.

Harris J. It's not NICE to discriminate. *J Med Ethics.* 2005; 31: 373–5.

Ministry of Justice. *Deprivation of Liberty Safeguards: Code of Practice.* London: Ministry of Justice; 2008. Available at: www.dh.gov.uk/en/Publicationsandstatistics/Publications/PublicationsPolicyAndGuidance/DH_085476 (accessed 15 April 2009).

National Institute for Health and Clinical Excellence. *donepezil, Galantamine, rivastigmine (review) and memantine for the treatment of Alzheimer's disease.* Technology Appraisal Guidance No. 111. London: NIHCE; 2007. Available at: www.nice.org.uk/Guidance/TA111 (accessed 15 April 2009).

National Institute for Health and Clinical Excellence and Social Care Institute for Excellence. *Dementia: supporting people with dementia and their carers in health and social care.* NICE Clinical Guideline 42. London: NIHCE; 2006. Available at: www.nice.org.uk/Guidance/CG42 (accessed 15 April 2009).

Post SG. Alzheimer's disease: ethics and progression of dementia. *Clin Geriatr Med.* 1994; 10: 379–94.

Post SG, Whitehouse PJ. Fairhill Guidelines on ethics of the care of people with Alzheimer's disease: a clinical summary. *J Am Geriatr Soc.* 1995; 43: 1423–9.

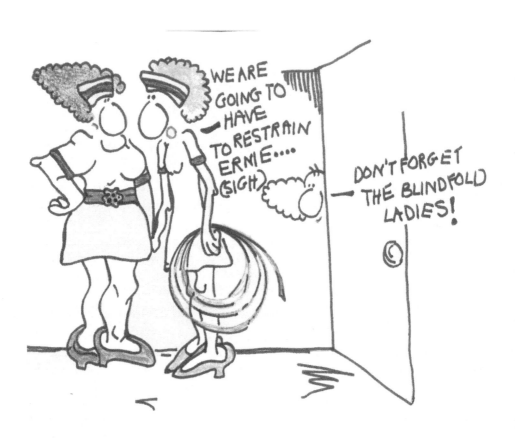

CHAPTER 13

The lawful use of restraints

Gwen M Sayers and Gurcharan S Rai

INTRODUCTION

Restraining a competent person without consent is unlawful and constitutes a criminal assault; therefore restraining one who lacks capacity to consent requires sound justification. Restraining individuals reduces their autonomy and limits their choices. They are prevented from pursuing their own good in their own manner. Yet John Stuart Mill, who so described this fundamental freedom in his essay 'On Liberty',[1] accorded it only to competent individuals rather than those who, in the care of others, required protection from injury to themselves and injury to others.

There is evidence that the use of restraints increases in direct proportion to the age of the patient and the level of cognitive impairment, regardless of the setting.[2] Restraint may be physical or chemical, but the underlying assumptions are those articulated by Mill – confused patients are restrained for their own benefit or the benefit of others. The flip side of these benefits is the damage that is undoubtedly caused by restraint, both by reducing the dignity of patients and exposing them to the risk of adverse physical effects. Hence, as in other areas of ethics, before a decision is taken to restrain a patient, a benefit/burden equation needs to be balanced. Further, the way in which the equation is balanced should be compatible with recent changes in English law.

CASE 13.1

Mrs A, an 86-year-old woman with dementia, is admitted to a general medical ward with pneumonia that is successfully treated. Although she has recovered, her discharge is delayed because she is unable to care for herself. While awaiting institutional placement, her behaviour becomes problematic. She tends to sleep

---

during the day and is noisy and aggressive at night when she wanders and climbs into other patients' beds. There are fewer nurses on the night shift and they struggle to provide the amount of supervision required by Mrs A. They therefore ask the doctors to prescribe night-time sedation. The sedation is cumulative and the patient now sleeps both day and night. Consequently her food and fluid intake declines. One morning she is unable to be aroused. Blood tests show that the serum sodium level is 181 mmol/l. Although she is treated with intravenous fluids, she dies soon after without regaining consciousness.

There are good moral arguments supporting aversion to restraint. Dodds argues that respect for autonomy is a duty that persists, and is thus owed even to those who lack legal capacity. She therefore believes that there is only limited justification for restraining patients on paternalistic grounds.[3] There are equally sound clinical reasons to avoid restraining frail elderly people, because of risks associated with their use (*see* Table 13.1).

TABLE 13.1 Risks associated with use of restraints

Injuries from falls
Accidental death from strangulation
Decline in function
Skin breakdown
Cardiac stress
Reduced appetite
Dehydration
Emotional and behavioural problems

Source: Evans and Strumpf, op. cit.

The question of when, if ever, to restrain a confused elderly patient is therefore debatable. This chapter will outline situations where restraint may be necessary – when the benefits outweigh the harms – and describe safeguards to ensure that restraint is proportionate and justified.

Although restraint has been curtailed since 1987 in the USA, by the Nursing Home Reform Act as part of the Omnibus Budget Reconciliation Act (OMBRA), in the UK relevant legislation is fairly recent. The Human Rights Act 1998 (HRA) and the Mental Capacity Act 2005 (MCA) will be used to support an approach regarding whether and when restraint is lawful.

THE USE OF RESTRAINT

Elderly patients in hospital wards and nursing homes are in an unfamiliar environment shared with strangers. They may be prone to disorientation, which can manifest as disturbed behaviour, especially if they are cognitively impaired, acutely ill or on medication. Discomfort (due to pain, constipation or a full bladder) may cause attempts to wander, or boredom may prompt a wish to escape. Many of these patients may be unsteady, have poor vision and be likely to fall. Falls can result in serious injuries, notably fractured hips and subdural haematomata, either of which can cause death. Therefore staff, afraid of being charged with a breach of their duty of care, may use restraint as a defensive measure.

Three main types of restraint are used within an institutional setting.

1 *Restraints that limit mobility*

Restraints that prevent free mobility include bedrails that hinder patients trying to leave the bed, and chairs with trays that entrap patients in a seated position. Bedrails, however, are not necessarily a deterrent to patients determined to climb out of bed. If a confused patient manages to scale them, the rails increase the height of the fall thereby increasing the damage sustained. All forms of restraint resulting in immobility take their toll by causing loss of muscle strength and a predisposition towards the development of pressure sores. Therefore, measures implemented to protect the patient from the risk of falling may lead to greater, though different, dangers.

2 *Restraints that prevent access to one's body*

Restraints that prevent patients from accessing their own bodies include tying patients' limbs or using glove mittens. Such restraints are used to facilitate the administration of medication, to prevent patients dislodging nasogastric tubes and other internal lines, or to prevent self-harm. These restraints are now rarely used, both because they are degrading and because of their potential adverse effects. Patients may struggle against ties, resulting in abrasive skin injuries or even gangrene of a limb through disruption of blood supply.

3 *Chemical restraints*

Chemical restraints or sedating agents are used, especially on general wards, to contain noisy and disruptive patients or those with behavioural problems – largely for the sake of other patients. The use of major tranquillisers for patients suffering from dementia has been broadly condemned because of adverse effects. Apart from over-sedation as described in Case 13.1, these drugs have also been linked to increased cardiovascular mortality. Their other common side-effects, such as postural hypotension and extrapyramidal manifestations, increase the likelihood of falls. Moreover, these drugs can worsen confusional states, so magnifying the problem for which they were initially prescribed.

There is thus good reason to advocate zero tolerance of restraints. This ideal, however, would require resources in excess of those available within the National Health Service (NHS). For example, disruptive and aggressive patients nursed in side rooms with one-to-one care would not require sedating agents. Patients with internal lines would not dislodge them if watched constantly and discouraged from handling their tubes. Patients would not fall out of bed if nursed in a side room on a mattress placed on the floor.

Such measures are usually not possible because, except in intensive care settings or in psychiatric wards, the nurse-to-patient ratio makes close monitoring of all confused patients difficult if not impossible, especially at night. Side rooms are a scarce commodity that may be prioritised for patients with infectious diseases or dying patients who require privacy. The best alternative to prohibition of restraint is to adopt a high threshold to the use of restraint and develop a policy that ensures reasonable safeguards and appropriate justification for those cases where restraint appears to be the only safe option. The policy would have to comply with recent UK legislation.[4]

HUMAN RIGHTS ACT 1998

The HRA, which came into effect in 2000, made it unlawful for a public authority to act in a way that was incompatible with any of the articles incorporated in the European Convention on Human Rights. The term 'public authority' encompasses NHS Trusts as well as individual doctors who, in the course of their duties, treat patients within the remit of the Trusts. The articles relevant to restraint that will be considered are Articles 2, 3 and 8. Article 5 (right to liberty), which applies to individuals who are detained, falls outside the scope of this chapter.

Article 2: right to life

Article 2 imposes a strong duty on the state not to interfere with life, and a weaker duty to protect life. This implies a strict prohibition against causing death, without a correspondingly stringent obligation to preserve life at all costs. The European Court of Human Rights, by recognising a limitation on the obligation to preserve life, released authorities from an impossible or disproportionate burden.

This approach is echoed in common law and in guidance provided by the General Medical Council and the British Medical Association. Doctors are obliged to provide life-prolonging treatment only when it in the patient's best interests. Therefore, if continuing treatment is considered to be in an incompetent patient's best interests and the patient's life will be threatened if restraints are not used, the doctor may be obliged to restrain the patient in order to provide life-prolonging treatment.

CASE 13.2

Mr B, an acutely confused elderly man, has developed *C. difficile* following treatment of a urinary tract infection. He has profuse diarrhoea and requires medication and hydration. He, however, refuses oral intake and pulls out both nasogastric tubes and intravenous lines. His wife asks whether his hands can be immobilised so that treatment can be effectively administered in order to save his life. This is accomplished by using mittens. After a few days of treatment, his confusional state improves, the mittens are removed and oral fluids and medications are resumed. He is discharged home when well.

When treatment is both life-prolonging and in the patient's best interests, there would need to be strong justification for not using restraints if restraints are essential to treat. This is when Article 3 rights may be relevant.

Article 3: prohibition of torture

Sometimes two articles of the HRA, like two moral principles, can conflict. For example, we cannot always respect an individual patient's confidentiality when doing so threatens public interests. So it is with Articles 2 and 3. Although Article 2 confers a right to life, this right is not absolute. There are times when the nature of life-prolonging treatment may be disproportionately painful, or pointless if the benefits to be gained are short term. In such cases treatment, particularly if it requires restraint, may be at odds with Article 3 rights.

The full text of Article 3 is: 'No-one should be subjected to inhuman or degrading treatment or punishment.' On this basis, there could be argument for a blanket prohibition on restraint, so allowing Article 3 rights always to trump those conferred by Article 2. Restraint, however, when necessary medically and used in conformity with medical standards, has been deemed legally acceptable by the European Court of Human Rights; but the type of restraint, and the way in which it is used can breach Article 2 rights. Further, denial of treatment has, in itself, been found to amount to degrading treatment by the European Court.

In the UK, this ruling is echoed in common law. In the case of *Re MB*,[5] Butler-Sloss LJ said that, when treating an incompetent patient, doctors needed to judge in each case the degree of force or compulsion necessary. They had to balance whether to continue or discontinue forcibly imposed treatment.

Article 8: right to respect for private and family life

Article 8 rights cover the individual's physical integrity. This becomes particularly important when conflict arises between the relatives and the health professionals. In *Glass v UK*,[6] doctors withheld resuscitation and administered morphine to a severely disabled child, despite the mother's objections and without judicial authorisation. This treatment was found to breach Article 8 by interfering with the child's right to respect for physical integrity. The issue of whether the mother had Article 8 rights separate from those of the patient was not considered by the Court.

Thus, Human Rights law informs us that restraint, although degrading at face value, is acceptable when used (proportionately) in order to treat a patient who would otherwise have to forego beneficial treatment. This only applies when treatment provides a significant benefit such as life prolongation, or prevents a significant harm. It must be borne in mind that failure to treat in such cases may also be degrading. In the case of individuals who are not competent, the decision regarding treatment or withholding treatment should be discussed with relatives, and when disagreement arises there may be need for judicial review.

MENTAL CAPACITY ACT 2005

Whereas the HRA provides a broad brush approach to rights and freedoms, the MCA which came into force in 2007, is more specific in its directives. Prior to the MCA, in English law no person could provide or withhold proxy consent for an incompetent adult. Instead, doctors were authorised to treat such patients in their best interests on the basis of necessity. Therefore, in the case of restraints used to administer life-saving treatment, the clinical team would be authorised to make the decision, as described above in the case of *Re MB*. The MCA changes this by allowing a donor (the patient) to confer a lasting power of attorney on a donee with authority to make decisions concerning the patient's personal welfare.

Section 6 of the MCA defines restraint as either the use or threat of use of force in order to undertake an action that the patient resists, or restriction of the patient's freedom of movement whether or not the patient resists. Section 11 of the Act further imposes restrictions on the lasting power of attorney when it comes to restraint by requiring three conditions to be satisfied. These are:
1 the patient must lack capacity in relation to the matter in question
2 the donee must believe that the restraining act is necessary to prevent harm to the patient
3 the restraint must be a proportionate response to the likelihood of harm to the patient and the seriousness of the harm.

The MCA requires that all decisions made on behalf of incompetent people must be made in their best interests and takes a significant step towards empowering proxy decision makers to choose what constitutes the best interests of their loved ones. If there is no donee with lasting power of attorney, the MCA requires the clinical decision maker to take into account the views of anyone engaged in caring for the person, provided it is practical and appropriate to consult them. Therefore it is good practice to consult relatives whenever feasible before using restraints.

CASE 13.3

Mrs C, a patient in her nineties, who has dementia, is admitted to hospital with a fractured hip following a fall at the nursing home where she lives. She requires sedation in order to X-ray her hip and resists all attempts to draw blood or insert lines. The orthopaedic surgeon says that she is unlikely to survive an operation and recommends pain palliation. Her relatives believe that Mrs C has no quality of life and that surgery would be cruel. They say that she would refuse surgery if she was capable of deciding. Although able to swallow, Mrs C refuses food, fluids and oral medication. Restraining her in order to hydrate or nourish her is not thought to be in her best interests since her prospects for recovery are negligible. She is treated with pain-relieving patches and dies peacefully within a few days.

Deprivation of liberty is a wider encroachment on freedom than the shorter-term restriction of movement described above. The Bournewood case, in which a patient with severe learning difficulties was detained without eliciting the provisions of the Mental Health Act 1983, was found by the European Court of Human Rights to breach Article 5 (right to liberty and security). In order to address the vulnerability of severely incapacitated patients housed in hospital wards or nursing homes, the government has amended the MCA 2005 to include deprivation of liberty safeguards. These safeguards, implemented on 1 April 2009, will ensure that persons lacking the capacity to consent, who are at risk of being deprived of their liberty, are identified. Authorisation will then need to be obtained from the relevant local authority for those in care homes, or the Primary Care Trust, for those in hospital.[7]

GUIDELINES REGARDING RESTRAINT

All hospitals and nursing homes should have policies regarding restraint. When deciding whether or not to restrain a patient, the following factors should be considered.

1   Restraining a competent patient without their consent is unlawful.
2   When an incompetent patient requires medical treatment that can only be administered by using restraint, this is permissible provided:
    — the form of restraint used is the least restrictive possible and used for the shortest time possible
    — the treatment proposed must be in the patient's best interest

— the consequences of not treating will be seriously harmful to the patient

— restraint should be a short-term measure with the expectation of recovery

— restraint is practically possible.

3 When an incompetent patient cannot be safely nursed without restraint, this is permissible provided:

— the form of restraint used is the least restrictive possible and used for the shortest time possible

— all other avenues of nursing without restraint have been explored

— not restraining the patient will pose a serious threat to safety of the patient or of others.

4 In all cases where restraint is deemed necessary, assent should be sought from relatives. If the relatives refuse assent to restraint in order to administer life-prolonging treatment which the medical team believe is in the patient's best interest, a legal opinion should be sought.

5 In all cases where restraint is believed to be necessary, the reasons why restraint is used and with whom it was discussed should be carefully documented in the patient's notes.

KEY POINTS

- Restraining a competent person without consent is unlawful and constitutes a criminal assault.
- The Human Rights Act 1998 and the Mental Capacity Act 2005 are relevant to the use of restraints for patients who lack capacity to consent.
- Human rights law informs us that restraint, although degrading at face value, is acceptable when used (proportionately) in order to treat a patient who would otherwise have to forego beneficial treatment.
- Restraint, when medically necessary and used in conformity with medical standards, has been found to be legally acceptable by the European Court of Human Rights.
- Denial of treatment can also amount to degrading treatment in law.
- Section 6 of the MCA 2005 sets limitations on acts that involve restraint. Section 11 of the Act places restrictions on those with lasting powers of attorney who restrain, or authorise restraint of, a patient who lacks capacity.
- The Deprivation of Liberty Safeguards amendment to the MCA 2005 provides procedures for authorising the deprivation of liberty of adults who lack capacity to consent to being housed in hospitals and care homes.
- All hospitals and nursing homes should have policies regarding the use of restraints.

REFERENCES

1 Mill JS. *Three Essays: On Liberty; Representative Government; The Subjection of Women.* Oxford: Oxford University Press; 1975.

2 Evans LK, Strumpf NE. Tying down the elderly: a review of the literature on physical restraint. *J Am Geriatric Soc.* 1989; **37**: 65–74.

3 Dodds S. Exercising restraint: autonomy, welfare and elderly patients. *J Med Ethics.* 1996; **22**: 160–3.

4 Sayers GM, Gabe SM. Restraint in order to feed: justifying a lawful policy for the UK. *Euro J Health Law.* 2007; **14**: 3–20.

5 *Re MB* (Medical Treatment) [1997] 2 FLR 426.

6 *Glass v United Kingdom* (2004) Application No. 61827/00.

7 www.dh.gov.uk/en/Publicationsandstatistics/Publications/PublicationsPolicyAnd Guidance/DH_085476

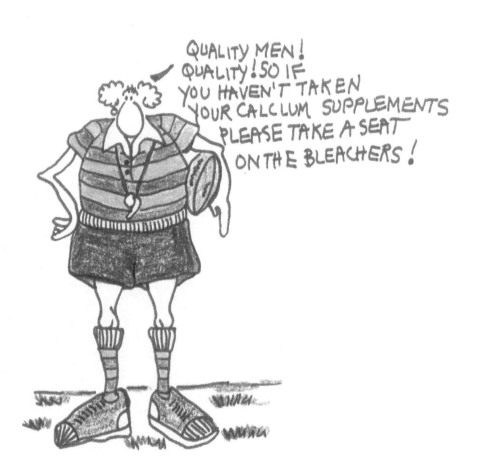

CHAPTER 14

Quality of life in healthcare decisions

Ann Bowling

INTRODUCTION: QUALITY OF LIFE VERSUS LENGTH OF LIFE

Research in the USA indicates that patients have expressed a preference for survival for a shorter life of improved quality.[1,2] However, research on cancer patients in the UK has shown that most patients would accept toxic chemotherapy for minimal benefit in relation to prolongation of life.[3] Similarly, newly admitted in-patients under and over age 65, with acute coronary syndrome, reported that they would accept any treatment, however extreme, to return to their former health.[4] Research in the USA has also shown that most patients in geriatric wards indicated that they wanted to be resuscitated if their heart stopped beating, while few of their doctors had marked them for resuscitation in the medical notes.[5] It appears that doctors often rate the quality of life of the patient as lower than the patient perceives it, and the life itself of lower value than the patient rates it. The only way to face ethical dilemmas about treatments is to ask the patient about their perception of their quality of life and their treatment preferences.

AGE-RELATED TREATMENT POLICIES

Negative assumptions about the quality of life of elderly people, together with a general ageism in Western society, have led to age cut-off points for treatments, which are not based on the evidence of clinical effectiveness, in some health districts. This is apparent, for example, in cardiology in relation to access to rehabilitation centres, cardiological investigations and specific, clinically effective treatments (e.g. revascularisation through coronary artery bypass graft (CABG)).[6,7]

However, increasingly the literature on health-related quality of life does not justify age-related policies. For example, a five-year follow-up study of the broader quality of life of 1371 patients aged over 74 years at operation (mean age at operation 77 years) and 257 'neutral-risk' patients (mean age at operation 58 years), all of whom were undergoing CABG, reported that CABG is justified in very elderly people because the health-related quality of the extended survival was as good as that reported for younger patients and that for age-adjusted populations.[8] Although few clinical trials of treatments currently include patients aged over 65 or 70 years, it is important to measure the effects of treatments in older people as well as in younger subjects. This is more pertinent with the ageing of the population, and evidence of a healthier older population than in the past, together with the emphasis on positive ageing and equal rights to appropriate and clinically effective treatments among all age groups.

Although over-investigation and medical intervention to prolong life at the expense of quality of life at any age merit ethical debate, and while any mortality risk must be balanced against the potential gains in life years and in quality of life, it is important to ensure equal access to clinically effective and appropriate treatments from which older as well as younger people can benefit in the broadest sense.

MEASURING HEALTH-RELATED QUALITY OF LIFE

Such studies indicate the value of measuring health-related quality of life when assessing the outcome of clinical interventions. The broader measurement of health outcome has become a cornerstone of health services research. Purchasers of healthcare want to know what health gain interventions provide. This emphasis is positive, and health-related quality of life assessment is increasingly incorporated into criteria for the assessment of people's needs for effective services. Treatments and interventions need to be evaluated in terms of whether they are more likely to lead to an outcome of a life worth living in social, psychological and physical terms, and people themselves are the best judges of this in relation to their own lives.

Health-related quality of life is a subjective concept, and relates to the perceived effects of health status on the ability to live a fulfilling life. This encompasses functional ability in relation to ability to perform self-care tasks, domestic tasks and mobility, role functioning (e.g. ability to function in work, social roles such as parenting, etc.), the existence and quality of relationships and social interaction, psychological well-being (e.g. life satisfaction, adjustment, coping ability), autonomy and control, and mental health (e.g. anxiety, depression, cognitive state). As with the concept, the potential range of dimensions of health-related quality of life which could be measured in studies of health outcomes is wide. A population survey of people aged 65 years that asked them how they perceived quality of life reported that they emphasised psychological characteristics (e.g. outlook on life), health and functional ability, social relationships, neighbourhood (e.g. safety, facilities, transport), having enough money and retaining their independence.[9] Individualised measures are more complex to analyse than standardised questionnaires and scales, but they are invaluable where there is uncertainty about whether all relevant questions have been included in a questionnaire, and for informing the items (questions) that make up scales and enhancing their content validity. For example, respondents' detailed statements about quality of life in the former study were used to form Likert scale ('Strongly agree' to 'Strongly disagree') statements for the multi-dimensional Older People's Quality of Life Questionnaire, which the author is currently testing with three national samples of older people, and with good results to date.

On a day-to-day basis, quality of life on the ward may have to be based on subjective assessment, taking into account what the patient thinks, and his or her morale, ability to communicate, mental capacity, degree of incontinence and physical dependency. For example, a person with end-stage dementia who cannot recognise their loved ones can be assumed to have reached a stage where, to that person, the meaning of human life has deteriorated, and they therefore have a poor quality of life.

As Elder[10] pointed out, common justifications for inequitable treatment of older people are perceived lack of benefit, the belief that treatments for older people represent an inappropriate use of scarce resources and the misconception that patients do not want more invasive treatments. He argued that clinicians do not need to know if an older person will benefit more or less than a younger person from a specific treatment, but rather whether a patient of any age will benefit more from a specific treatment compared with usual care. The justification of inequity with reference to the appropriate use of resources by age of patient has been reinforced by health policy decisions (e.g. the UK's National Institute for Health and Clinical Excellence) using quality-adjusted life years (QALYs), which are inherently ageist.

CHOOSING A MEASURE OF HEALTH-RELATED QUALITY OF LIFE

When choosing a health-related quality-of-life measure, or a battery of measures, key questions to consider are whether a generic or disease-specific measure is needed, and whether this should be supplemented with more detailed domain-specific measures (e.g. depression scales) that are important to the aims of the study. The type of scale and domain-specific scales will vary according to the type of patient under study.

Generic measures usually tap social, psychological and physical areas of life. They are used for population health profiles and in order to make comparisons with other conditions (e.g. outcome of treatments for different conditions). The latter are useful when comparisons of the costs of treatments in relation to their benefits (outcomes) are required.

POPULAR MEASUREMENT SCALES

One of the most popular, concise generic measures is the Short Form 36-item Health Survey Questionnaire (SF-36).[11] This is also often used as a core component to facilitate comparisons across populations in disease-specific batteries of measures. These need to be interviewer administered to obtain the best item response rates among elderly people.[12] In the USA, a commonly used generic scale developed for use with elderly people is the Older Americans' Resources and Services Schedule (OARS), although the full instrument is lengthy.[13]

Because of the multiple morbidity that is often found in older people, and potential effects on physical functioning, emotional well-being and mental state, most investigators prefer to use a battery of pertinent domain-specific scales when evaluating the health status or health outcomes of elderly people. These may be used together with relevant disease-specific or generic measures, while bearing in mind the need to limit respondent fatigue. Popular domain-specific scales include Lawton's (1975) Philadelphia Geriatric Center Morale Scale,[14] the Abbreviated Mental Test (AMT)[15] and the Geriatric Depression Scale (GDS).[16] A concise measure of anxiety and depression, which does not include somatic items and is therefore appropriate for use with older people, is the Hospital Anxiety and Depression Scale (HADS).[17] The Barthel Index[18] is often used to measure physical functioning, but this is only suitable for severely ill, institutionalised populations. It focuses on self-care at the expense of instrumental tasks of daily living (e.g. domestic tasks) and wider physical mobility. The functioning sub-section of the OARS is superior to most scales for use with elderly people.

There is no consensus on recommended batteries of scales. More recently there has been an emphasis on also asking people to list themselves what areas of their life are most important or which have been most affected by their condition. Given that people will have different priorities in life (e.g. the ability to go up a flight of stairs is less important to someone who does not have stairs), these newer instruments provide the means by which individuality can be assessed scientifically.[19,20]

CRITERIA FOR SCALE DEVELOPMENT AND FOR SELECTING A SCALE

The criteria for measurement scales or batteries of scales are listed below.[21] When reviewing scales for use, potential users should check the scale's literature for information on each of these areas, and use an appropriate scale where this information is satisfactory.

Conceptual and measurement model

The conceptual and empirical basis for combining multiple items into a single scale score(s) should be provided. Descriptive statistics for each scale should be provided by scale developers (frequencies, means, central tendency and dispersion, skewness and frequency of missing data), as should procedures for weighting and scoring.

Reliability

The instrument should be free from random error and therefore homogenous in content (high correlations between items and tests of internal consistency). It should be reproducible over time (where changes in scores are not expected) and between raters at one point in time. Scale developers should provide a clear description of the methods used to test for reliability, by type of population, and information on the results of tests for reliability.

Validity

This is the degree to which an instrument measures what it purports to measure. The scale developer should provide evidence that the content of the scale is appropriate and relevant to its intended use, that its construct is sound and that it correlates with measures with which it is theoretically expected to correlate, and that it correlates with a criterion measurement ('gold standard'). As with reliability, full details of the methods, samples and results of tests of validity should be provided by the developer.

Responsiveness

This is the sensitivity of the instrument to true change (e.g. in the patient's condition). This is assessed in before/after studies of interventions and a comparison of scale scores. Assessment of responsiveness involves estimation of the effect size. This is an estimate of the magnitude of change in health status, and it translates the before/after changes into a standard unit of measurement. Scale developers should provide information on responsiveness from longitudinal study data on clearly defined populations.

Interpretability

This is the degree to which meaning can be assigned to the scale's scores. It can be provided by comparative data on the distribution of scores in different populations and on the relationship of scores to clinically recognised conditions and outcomes (including predictive ability of the score in relation to death). The scale developer should provide details of the populations to whom the scale was administered and descriptive statistics.

Burden

Respondent burden can be defined as the time, energy and other demands placed on the respondents during the completion of the instrument. Administrative burden is the demand placed on those who administer it. Developers should not place undue strain on the respondent during the completion of their instruments, and should provide information on average completion times, comprehension or reading levels required, interviewer training required, and the acceptability of the instrument (e.g. indicated by the level of missing data and refusal rates plus reasons).

Alternative forms

These include all of the modes of administration of an instrument, such as self-completion, observer ratings, interviewer-administered and computer-assisted completion. Evidence of reliability, validity, responsiveness, interpretability and burden should be provided for each form of the instrument.

Cultural and language adaptations

The scale developer should provide information about the conceptual equivalence (equivalence of relevance and meaning of the same concepts) and linguistic equivalence (equivalence of question wording and meaning in the formulation of items, response choices) of the scale in the different languages and repeat the evaluations of its measurement properties (reliability, validity, responsiveness, interpretability and burden). The scale developer should provide evidence of the methods used to achieve equivalence (e.g. assessment within each cultural or language group to which the instrument will be applied, two forward translations from the source language by experienced translators and health status research, resulting in a pooled forward translation; backward translations to the source language resulting in a pooled translation; review of translations by lay and expert panels, with revisions and field testing to provide evidence of comparability and explanation of any differences).

These criteria should be used to evaluate the strengths and weaknesses of measurement instruments. A wide range of generic and disease-specific measurement scales were concisely reviewed by Bowling in 2001[12] and 2005.[22]

KEY POINTS

- People themselves are the best judges of an outcome of 'life worth living'.
- The only way to address an ethical dilemma about treatment is to ask the patient about their perception of their quality of life and their preferences.
- If the patient is not competent to answer this question, then ask their next of kin or carer who knows them best.
- In the ward setting, quality of life may have to be assessed after taking into

account the views of the patient and their carers with regard to morale, their symptoms as well as their physical dependency, their mental capacity and whether they are incontinent.

● Although there is no consensus on the recommended battery of scales, commonly used instruments include Lawton's Philadelphia Geriatric Morale Scale, the Abbreviated Mental Test and the Geriatric Depression Scale.

REFERENCES

1 McNeil BJ, Weichselbaum R, Pauker SG. Fallacy of the five-year survival in lung cancer. *NEJM.* 1978; **299**: 1397–401.

2 McNeil BJ, Weichselbaum R, Pauker SG. Speech and survival: trade-offs between quality and quantity of life in laryngeal cancer. *NEJM.* 1981; **305**: 982–7.

3 Slevin ML, Stubbs L, Plant HJ, *et al.* Attitudes to chemotherapy: comparing views of patients with cancer with those of doctors, nurses and the general public. *BMJ.* 1990; **300**: 1458–60.

4 Bowling A, Culliford L, Smith D, *et al.* What do patients really want? Patients' preferences for treatment for angina. *Health Expectations.* 2008; **11**: 137–47.

5 Liddle J, Gilleard C, Neil A. Elderly patients' and their relatives' views on CPR [letter]. *Lancet.* 1993; **342**: 1055.

6 Bowling A, Bond M, McClay M, *et al.* Equity in access to exercise tolerance testing, coronary angiography, and coronary artery bypass grafting by age, sex and clinical indications. *Heart.* 2001; **85**: 680–6.

7 Collinson J, Bakhai A, Flather MD, *et al.* The management and investigation of elderly patients with acute coronary syndromes without ST elevation: an evidence-based approach? Results of the Prospective Registry of Acute Ischaemic Syndromes in the UK (PRAIS-UK). *Age Ageing.* 2005; **34**: 61–6.

8 Walter PJ, Mohan R. Health-related quality of life in octogenarians 5 years after coronary bypass surgery. *Qual Life Res.* 1994; **3**: 63.

9 Bowling A, Gabriel Z, Dykes J, *et al.* Let's ask them: a national survey of definitions of quality of life and its enhancement among people aged 65 and over. *Int J Ageing Hum Dev.* 2003; **56**: 269–306.

10 Elder AT. Which benchmarks for age discrimination in acute coronary syndrome? *Age Ageing.* 2005; **34**: 4–5.

11 Ware JE, Snow KK, Kosinski M, *et al.* SF-36 Health Survey: manual and interpretation guide. Boston, MA: The Health Institute, New England Medical Center; 1993.

12 Bowling A. *Measuring Disease: a review of disease-specific quality-of-life measurement scales.* 2nd ed. Buckingham: Open University Press; 2001.

13 Fillenbaum GG, Smyer MA. The development, validity and reliability of the OARS Multidimensional Functional Assessment Questionnaire. *J Gerontol.* 1981; **36**: 428–34.

14 Lawton MP. The Philadelphia Geriatric Morale Scale: a revision. *J Gerontol.* 1975; **30**: 85–9.

15 Hodkinson HM. Evaluation of a mental test score for assessment of mental impairment in the elderly. *Age Ageing.* 1972; **1**: 233–8.

16 Ysavage JA, Brink TL, Rose TL, *et al.* Development and validation of a geriatric depression screening scale: a preliminary report. *J Psychiatr Res.* 1983; **17**: 37–49.

17 Zigmond AS, Snaith RP. The Hospital Anxiety and Depression Scale. *Acta Psychiatr Scand.* 1983; **67**: 361–70.

18 Mahoney FI, Barthel DW. Functional evaluation: the Barthel Index. *Maryland State Med J.* 1965; **14**: 61–5.

19 O'Boyle CA, McGee H, Hickey A, *et al.* Reliability and validity of judgement analysis as a method for assessing quality of life. *Br J Clin Pharmacol.* 1989; **27**: 155.

20 Bowling A. The effects of illness on quality of life: findings from a survey of households in Great Britain. *J Epidemiol Com Health.* 1996; **50**: 149–55.

21 Medical Outcomes Trust. Source pages. In: *Products, Applications, Services: a resource directory for the health outcomes field.* Boston, MA: Medical Outcomes Trust; 1996.

22 Bowling A. *Measuring Health: a review of quality-of-life measurement scales.* 3rd ed. Buckingham: Open University Press; 2005.

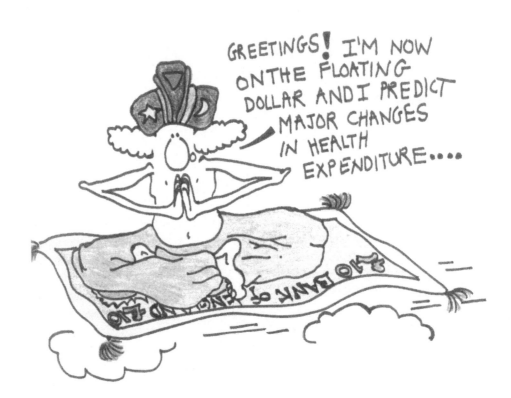

CHAPTER 15

Ethical issues and expenditure on health and social care

Steven Luttrell

THE NATIONAL HEALTH SERVICE

In the early part of the twentieth century, medical services in the UK were spread unevenly and large numbers of poor people were not covered by the National Insurance Scheme. The National Health Service (NHS) was established to provide equitable healthcare provision according to need, irrespective of wealth or geographical location. Over time, it became increasingly clear that comprehensive care, free at the point of delivery, was politically unsustainable. Prescription charges were introduced in 1951, and charges for ophthalmic and dental treatments were introduced thereafter. One of the most radical assaults on the provision of comprehensive care was the shedding by the NHS of substantial parts of its previously held responsibilities for continuing care. In 1982, the NHS was providing 75% of long-stay care for people aged 75 years and over. In 1996 this was reduced to just 18%. During the same time period the population of people aged 75 years and over increased by 25%.

HEALTHCARE OR SOCIAL CARE?

The starting point for any discussion on the economics of healthcare must be a consideration of the meaning of the term 'healthcare'. To define certain care needs as social rather than health related transfers the funding of such services from the NHS (where, in general, costs are provided for) to social services (where, in general, costs are means tested). Although there are many areas of care which are agreed to fall clearly within the remit of the health service, there are others where this is not so obvious. For example, there has been substantial debate over which aspects of continuing care of people with disabilities should be regarded as healthcare and which should be regarded as social care. This debate was set on a legal footing in *R v North and East Devon Health Authority ex part Coughlan* (2000) All ER 850, which clarified the responsibilities of both healthcare and social care services in the provision of longer-term care for people with disabilities and continuing healthcare needs.

PRINCIPLES FOR RATIONING

No matter how narrowly healthcare is defined, there remains a widespread belief that demand for services exceeds supply, and that some form of rationing or prioritisation is necessary. Rationing of healthcare is by no means a new concept. For many decades the rationing of state-funded healthcare in the UK was undertaken either implicitly by clinicians in line with unwritten customs and practice or more explicitly by the application of controls on the supply of healthcare services and the creation of waiting lists and access barriers. Broadly speaking, healthcare has in the past been rationed according to need, ability to benefit, age and desert.

Need

The allocation of funds according to need has been a traditional function of the NHS. Initial formulas based on mortality ratios were used as proxies for need in order to redistribute funds. Empirical data have led to new formulas which are thought to be more sensitive to the influence of socio-economic factors on health, and which have been applied to the greater part of the NHS budget. However, it has been suggested that the marginal increase in equity associated with the use of the more recent formulas is probably very small, and that in future attention should be focused on the distribution of resources at local levels. Moreover, the allocation of funds according to need does not necessarily mean that such funds will confer benefit.

Ability to benefit

Utilitarian philosophy suggests that funds should be used to provide maximum benefit. It is argued that the use of effectiveness data alone perpetuates the inefficient use of resources and that rationing in healthcare must be informed by knowledge of the costs and consequences of alternative interventions. Over recent years there has been a growth in the number of interventions to which cost–benefit analysis has been applied. However, while the Department of Health has indicated that resources should increasingly be channeled towards those interventions which are known to be effective, the paucity of data on effectiveness and cost continues to create substantial difficulties for Primary Care Trusts. In addition, health services have generally been slow to implement changes in practice in response to new scientific evidence of treatment benefit.

Since 2000, the NHS has introduced a range of National Service Frameworks (NSFs) and published a large quantity of guidance through the National Institute for Health and Clinical Excellence (NICE) to encourage the faster implementation of clinical services and treatments where there is evidence of cost effectiveness. However, these systems have tended to work through pri-oritisation (more effective practice being encouraged) rather than rationing (less effective practice being stopped) and NICE has been criticised for overly concentrating on new and expensive treatments. It is also fair to say that while most evaluations have focused on the costs and benefits to health and health services, there is an increasing need to assess the costs and benefits to the social care sector arising from the application of healthcare interventions.

More recently, Primary Care Trusts in England have used national programme budgeting data to compare spending on services relative to other localities with similar geographical characteristics. This is a system which has informed the reallocation of resources by enabling resources to be released from services of little value and reallocated to newer and more effective services.

Age

In the past, healthcare has been extensively rationed by age. There is evidence that older people have been discriminated against with regard to renal replace-ment therapy, cardiological interventions and cancer treatments. A variety of reasons have been proposed to justify or explain this position.

1 It has been assumed that the needs of older people were somehow less important and that they would not, in any event, benefit from aggressive medical treatment. However, there is now a substantial body of scientific evidence suggesting that older people benefit from many medical interven-tions to which they would previously have been denied access (e.g. treatment of hypertension, thrombolysis for myocardial infarction, carotid artery sur-gery and renal replacement therapy). Increasingly it has been demonstrated that those populations at highest risk of death or complications are often the groups that benefit most from interventions. Thus in certain situations older patients, who are at a greater risk of death or morbidity than younger patients, benefit more from medical treatment.

2 It has been suggested that a strictly utilitarian method of allocating resources discriminates against older people. If it is assumed that the prime function of the NHS is to maximise health, and the 'quality-adjusted life year' (QALY) is used as a method of assessing outcome, then it becomes obvious that older people, with a shorter life expectancy, will generally rank lower on the prior-ity list than younger people. NICE has been criticised by some for placing a heavy reliance on the use of QALYs in its evaluations.

Harris argues against such a method of distributing resources, stating that patients want the opportunities to have the best possible combination of quantity and quality of life available to them, given their personal health status.[1] It may be valid to use outcome measures when choosing between rival therapies, but this system should not be used for allocating resources between different groups of patients. Harris believes that it is an integral part of distributive justice that people's moral claims to resources are not diminished by who they are (how young or old, rich or poor, powerful or weak they are) or by the quality of their lives. He argues that if the purpose of the NHS is to give people the services that they want for themselves, then they would be unlikely to choose the utilitarian approach. This argument has widespread appeal.

3 It is argued by some that the older you are, the more likely you are to have had your 'fair innings', and that it would be inequitable to deny a younger person benefit in order to provide benefit for an older person.

According to one view, the fair innings argument is based on the concept of an ideal life and the notion that individuals themselves reach a point in time when they have done all that they would have wished and feel that it is appropriate that they should now die. Although this is an argument which underpins the need for a system where patient autonomy is respected, it adds little to the debate about rationing healthcare.

According to another view, it is argued that resources should be rationed on the basis of the quality and length of life which any individual has already had. Those who have already had sufficient life of sufficient quality are of lower priority than those who have not. But how can one measure the total quality of any life and how should one decide where the cut-off point for a fair innings should be? A simpler approach has been to argue that resources should be rationed only according to the length of life which an individual has already had. This approach has popular appeal, as evidenced by the frequent media items concerning the plight of babies and children. However, it does highlight basic questions about the value that society attaches to any particular group of individuals. It might be that, despite popular appeal, to stigmatise and undervalue older people in favour of the young is detrimental to the fabric of society as a whole, especially a society that is founded on democratic principles where the value of one person is cherished as much as that of any other. The increasing political power of older people alongside the development of human rights law has done much in recent years to change society's attitude to age. Within the UK, the most explicit step to remove rationing on the basis of age was taken with the introduction of the National Service Framework for Older People, the first standard of which sets out a commitment and lists steps to remove ageism from health and social welfare decisions.

Desert

Giving less to those who are to blame for their illness has an instant emotional appeal. However, as a method for rationing healthcare it is flawed. It is very difficult to draw up a list of those illnesses to which a voluntary choice of life-style has contributed. Although alcoholism and cigarette smoking cause a host of illnesses, it is arguable that neither is a purely voluntary activity. If cigarette smoking is to be regarded as worthy of moral blame, then is eating an unhealthy diet to be similarly considered? Moreover, although the allocation of moral blame may fall within the responsibility of a legal system, it is questionable whether such judgments fall within the remit of a health service.

INTERNATIONAL MECHANISMS FOR RATIONING HEALTHCARE

A number of countries have taken steps to develop explicit guidelines about allocating health resources. Many have rejected a strictly utilitarian approach whereby services are ranked according to cost–benefit analysis.

The Swedish Commission stated that such considerations of efficiency should be limited to choices between different kinds of treatment for the same condition, and should not be invoked in the choice between claims for differ-ent services or specialities. It highlighted that all people have the same rights irrespective of their personal characteristics, resources should be devoted to those in greatest need and the most vulnerable groups should be given special consideration.

The Dunning Committee in the Netherlands recommended that all claims have to pass four tests: (i) is the intervention necessary to allow the individual to function in society? (ii) is the treatment effective? (iii) is the treatment efficient? (iv) could the treatment be considered a matter of individual responsibility?

In New Zealand, resource constraints are expressly recognised in the funding framework, the New Zealand Public Health and Disability Act 2000, the objec-tives of which include a population health focus, community participation and access to appropriate, effective and timely services.

Probably the most adventurous project for rationing healthcare evolved in the state of Oregon in the USA. Like every other US state, it had previously pro-vided only the poorest citizens with Medicaid and left a large percentage of the population unable to use medical services. The Oregon Health Plan was created in 1989 to expand coverage to citizens who at the time had no health insurance. However, in order to fund this expansion the state decided to ration healthcare in a transparent manner by introducing a prioritised list of treatments. A com-mission was set up to develop this list and heard evidence from both lay people and professionals. A line was drawn on the list based on the amount of money the state has set aside for its health plan. Everything above the line was covered but those treatments below the line were not. While the plan was initially viewed as successful and the numbers of uninsured people fell, conflicts arose between the state and federal government around the cuts caused by continually raising the 'line'. Moreover, the approach failed to control costs associated with the provision of those treatments above the line. Over the past decade, rates of the uninsured have returned close to the level they were at prior to the creation of the plan, prompting new proposals to reform health provision in 2007 which include universal coverage for children and a focus on cost control.

Rudolph Klein has suggested that the international principles on which there is agreement are too general to provide any assistance to those who are trying to create a core health service, and he states that rationing by such means has a trivial effect.[2] He believes instead that the reality of rationing is the numerous day-to-day decisions made by clinicians in the light of available resources and the circumstances of the patients before them.

The UK Government has not taken steps to define in explicit terms the principles which should be used to ration healthcare, appearing to rely instead on the development of policy from various NHS quality initiatives in combination with the accumulated decisions of healthcare trusts and individual clinicians. Much media and political attention has been paid to the fact that treatment options appear to differ from one part of the country to another. The mechanisms which have been established to counteract this include the development of national standards through a combination of National Service Frameworks and guidance set out by NICE. At the same time, the government has been keen to devolve responsibility for resource allocation to a local level, and responsibility for the allocation of over 70% of the NHS budget now rests with Primary Care Trusts. There are inevitable tensions created by a system which sets national standards but expects local financial responsibility. While these tensions have been masked by the recent expansion of the total NHS budget, any future tightening of total health spending may bring them into full view.

KEY POINTS

- The NHS was founded on the principle that it would provide an equitable system of healthcare.
- Narrowing the remit of the NHS has been used as a political method for reducing healthcare expenditure.
- Even if healthcare is defined in narrow terms, there appears to be a substantial financial gap between supply and demand.
- Rationing has traditionally been implicit and based on a variety of factors, such as need, ability to benefit, age and desert.
- A number of countries have attempted to make explicit the principles which should be used in rationing healthcare.
- In the UK, systems have been introduced over the past few years in order

to steer service delivery along lines which are backed by evidence of effectiveness.

● There is little international agreement about the most effective and fair methods of resource allocation.

REFERENCES

1 Harris J. Maximising the health of the whole community. The case against: what the principal objective of the NHS should really be. BMJ. 1997; **314**: 669–72.
2 Klein R. Defining a package of healthcare services the NHS is responsible for. The case against. BMJ. 1997; **314**: 506–9.

FURTHER READING

Alakeson V. Why Oregon went wrong. BMJ. 2008; **337**: 900–1.

Department of Health. NHS continuing health care: NHS and local council's responsibilities. HSC 2001/015: LAC (2001)18.

Department of Health. National Service Framework for Older People. London: Department of Health; 2001.

Doyal L. The rationing debate. Rationing within the NHS should be explicit: the case for. BMJ. 1997; **314**: 1114–180.

Drummond M. Economic evaluation of health interventions. BMJ. 2008; **337**: 770–1.

Government Committee on Choices in Healthcare. Report. Rijswijk, Netherlands: Ministry of Welfare, Health and Cultural Affairs; 1992.

Ham C. Retracing the Oregon trail: the experience of rationing and the Oregon health plan. BMJ. 1998; **316**: 1965–9.

Harris J. Unprincipled QALYs: a response to Cubbon. J Med Ethics. 1991; **17**: 185–8.

Harris J. Maximising the health of the whole community. The case against: what the principal objective of the NHS should really be. BMJ. 1997; **314**: 669–72.

House of Commons Health Committee. Priority Setting in the NHS: purchasing. Volume 1. London: HMSO; 1995.

Klein R. Defining a package of healthcare services the NHS is responsible for. The case against. BMJ. 1997; **314**: 506–9.

Manning J, Paterson J. Prioritization: rationing health care in New Zealand. J Law Med Ethics. 2005; **33**: 681–97.

Maynard A, Bloar K. Help or hindrance? The role of economics in rationing health care. Br Med Bull. 1995; **51**: 854–68.

Maynard A. Distributing healthcare rationing and the role of the physician in the United Kingdom National Health Service. In: A Grubb, MJ Mehlman, editors. Justice and Health Care: comparative perspectives. Chichester: John Wiley & Sons; 1995.

New B, on behalf of the Rationing Agenda Group. The rationing agenda in the NHS. BMJ. 1996; **312**: 1593–601.

Norheim O, Daniels M, Donaldson C, et al. Moving forward on rationing. BMJ. 2008; **337**: 903–6.

Sheldon T. Formula fever: allocating resources in the NHS. BMJ. 1997; **315**: 964.

Smith R. The failings of NICE. BMJ. 2000; **321**: 1363–4.

Swedish Parliamentary Priorities Commission. *Priorities in Healthcare.* Stockholm: Ministry of Health and Social Affairs; 1995.

Index

Entries in **bold** denote text in figures, tables or case examples.